Escape Fire

Donald M. Berwick

· ·

Introduction by Frank Davidoff, MD

Escape Fire

· ·

Designs for the
Future of Health Care

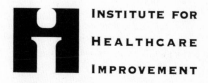

INSTITUTE FOR
HEALTHCARE
IMPROVEMENT

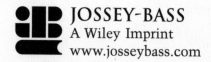

JOSSEY-BASS
A Wiley Imprint
www.josseybass.com

Published by Jossey-Bass
A Wiley Imprint
989 Market Street, San Francisco, CA 94103-1741   www.josseybass.com

Jossey-Bass books and products are available through most bookstores. To contact Jossey-
Bass directly, call our Customer Care Department within the U.S. at 800-956-7739,
outside the U.S. at 317-572-3986, or fax 317-572-4002.

Jossey-Bass also publishes its books in a variety of electronic formats. Some content that
appears in print may not be available in electronic books.

Library of Congress Cataloging-in-Publication Data

Berwick, Donald M. (Donald Mark), 1946–
    Escape fire: designs for the future of health care / Donald M. Berwick; introduction
by FrankDavidoff.
        p. ; cm.
    Keynote speeches presented at the annual National Forum on Quality Improvement
in Health Care, 1992–2002.
    Includes bibliographical references and index.
    ISBN 0-7879-7217-7
    1. Health care reform—United States. 2. Health services administration—United
States. 3. Medical care—United States—Quality control. 4. Patient advocacy—
United States.
    [DNLM: 1. Delivery of Health Care—trends—United States—Collected Works.
2. Organizational Innovation—United States—Collected Works. 4. Quality of Health
Care—trends—United States—Collected Works. W 84 AA1 B49e 2004] I. Institute
for Healthcare Improvement. National Forum. II. Title
RA395.A3B47 2004
362.1'0425—dc22   2003021193

Printed in the United States of America
FIRST EDITION
HB Printing   10 9 8 7 6 5 4 3 2 1

Contents

To Ann, with thanks, for love and courage

Preface

. . . .

To read these eleven speeches in one sitting, as I have now done, makes me dizzy. They pass before me at a speed disrespectful of the difficult decade they mark.

When I gave the first speech in this collection, "Kevin Speaks," in 1992 in front of sixteen hundred self-starting mavericks, the Institute for Healthcare Improvement was a young organization with a handful of employees, and health care had no quality movement at all. Ben, my oldest child, was a high school junior, and Becca, my youngest, was in first grade. (Ben is now a legislative aide on Capitol Hill and Becca is a high school senior.) Hillary Clinton was just about to try to rescue American health care. Avedis Donabedian and W. Edwards Deming were alive and well. So was my father. My family had not yet lived for a year in Alaska, or even imagined doing so. We were all healthy. I ran twenty miles a week, and my wife's two years of devastating illness were far in the future. The European Forum on Quality Improvement in Health Care and the Asia Pacific Forum did not exist. The Institute of Medicine (IOM) had no quality-of-care agenda on its screen. My hair was full and black.

Ten years later I gave the last speech in this collection, "Plenty," in a wholly different world. The National Forum on Quality Improvement in Health Care now had four thousand participants. A quality movement was expanding rapidly on at least three continents. The

Institute for Healthcare Improvement employed seventy people and worked with more than four hundred faculty members worldwide. The 8th European Forum on Quality Improvement in Health Care—with one thousand participants from forty-three nations— lay just ahead, and the 2nd Asia Pacific Forum—with seven hundred people from twenty-three nations—lay just behind. So did September 11. Harry Potter had met Voldemort, and my wife, Ann, was in her long convalescence, walking and working again. Avedis Donabedian, W. Edwards Deming, and Philip Berwick, my father, had been laid to rest, each after a long and difficult illness full of compassion from their caregivers and defects in their care. The IOM had spoken, in *To Err Is Human* and *Crossing the Quality Chasm:* "Between the health care we have and the health care we could have lies not just a gap, but a chasm." My right knee was totally blown and my jogging days were over. My hair had thinned and turned pure white.

With so much different, why do these speeches strike me as so repetitive? Metaphor after metaphor, list after list, story after story— but always the same. Year after year I can find only three messages at the core: *focus on the suffering, build and use knowledge,* and *cooperate.* There is no other suggestion in these pages—all else is fluff and padding, trying over and over again to make the signal comfortable enough to hear and eloquent enough to remember.

The words hide my impatience. Why is changing health care so hard?

Why don't we yet remember more reliably that our work has no other raison d'être than to relieve pain? In "Kevin Speaks" I wrote, "We are not here so that our organizations survive; we are here so that Kevin survives." Ten years later, recounting the story of a little girl, Alicia, who had cystic fibrosis, and her tireless father, Jim, I wrote, "We are here today for exactly—one reason—the same as Jim's—to make Alicia's senior prom night romantic."

Why are science and practice still so far apart? In 1993 I wrote, "The commitment to improving the match between scientific knowledge and actual practice, the commitment to 'appropriateness,' must come from the professionals whose actions constitute care"; and in 2001, "We need to get serious about promising every patient the benefit of care that draws on the best knowledge available anywhere."

Why do we continue trying to make great health care out of disconnected, separately perfected fragments instead of weaving the fabric of experience that our patients need from us? Kevin asked in 1992, "Do you ever talk to each other?" And a decade later I echoed him in my exhortation, "Cooperation is the highest professional value of all."

Though frustrated, I do find comfort in Joseph Juran's admonition, "The pace of change is majestic." From that higher perspective, improved results for the vast majority of patients still seem elusive; but the optimist in me thinks that something momentous—something substantial, meaningful, and rational—may have, after all, begun. I do sense a movement—not fast enough yet, but maybe a little "majestic." From a fringe collection of oddly placed provocateurs, the advocates of fundamentally changed health care have joined the mainstream. The IOM reports—*To Err Is Human* and *Crossing the Quality Chasm*—have chartered a whole new wave of scientifically grounded efforts to improve. A federal agency, the Agency for Healthcare Research and Quality (AHRQ), has changed its name to include "quality" and doubled its budget in pursuit of that aim. Big federal programs such as the Veterans Health Administration, the Bureau of Primary Health Care in the Health Resources and Services Administration, and Medicare have led the nation in embracing quality improvement aims. Patient safety, the cutting edge of quality, has front-page status. The Leapfrog Group—a progressive purchaser consortium in the United States—is trying to put quality criteria into health care contracting, making quality of care begin to seem like a serious business issue. Health care quality is now a major theme in medical literature, and both the *Joint Commission Journal* and the British Medical

Journal Publishing Group's journal *Quality and Safety in Health Care* are completely devoted to the issue. Training and residency programs are beginning to include quality and improvement in their required curricula for medical students. The National Health Service in the United Kingdom has established the Modernisation Agency, which now has eight hundred employees and massive improvement agendas, and is in the midst of the largest single-system improvement effort ever undertaken in any industry. Australia, New Zealand, and much of Scandinavia have all begun to place improvement of care at the center of their government-sponsored systems. The World Health Organization now has a chartering policy statement on patient safety from its 2002 World Health Assembly.

The change is preadolescent but massive. These eleven speeches punctuate a decade of stage setting, a getting-ready-to-change that in 1992 I could not even have begun to imagine. It would have seemed crazy even to hope for it.

Eleven National Forum speeches from now, how different will the message be? Now I can hope even more, without feeling crazy. The pedal point will be the same, of course: help people—every single person; use knowledge—all the knowledge; work together—cooperate, above all else. But maybe our hard work on these themes will at last have paid off so that new themes can also emerge out of results won, problems solved, and sensemaking returned.

In 2012—twenty years after "Kevin Speaks"—will a National Forum keynote speaker be fortunate enough to say that millions upon millions of patients—Kevin's successors—are safer, in less pain, more honored in their values and choices, wasting less time and money, and more confident in the reliability and gentleness of their care? Will we live longer and die less lonely and less afraid? Will we be able to celebrate that our health care remembers us in continuity, through our lives and across our communities, achieving well-being for populations as its measure of success rather than counting fragments and calling that "productivity"? Will we have replaced nineteenth-century information systems with twenty-first-century ones? Will we have restored joy in work for all professionals and staff, and be unembarrassed to say so? Will our young people, learning their craft, feel the highest sense of honor and delight in their choice of profession? Will we have come to think truly globally about the health we seek—for everyone—for all races, for all regions, for all nations?

Eleven speeches . . . a decade of change . . . a challenge defined . . . a movement well begun. Now, I'd say, things get *really* interesting.

September 2003   Donald M. Berwick, MD, MPP
                                                 Boston, Massachusetts

Acknowledgments

. . . .

The abundance I have found in colleagues and teachers awes me. At a very deep level, these speeches contain nothing original from me; they are more accurately recitations of lessons learned from others. The hundreds who have helped me will, I hope, excuse my mentioning by name only a few of the most central players in the phase of my career that this collection spans. Whatever expertise in technical improvement is mine comes from the patient and personal instruction of a generous, world-class varsity, including, among many others, Blan Godfrey, Kevin Nolan, Lloyd Provost, Jerry Langley, Ron Moen, Paul Plsek, Bob King, Ray Carey, Bob Lloyd, Jim Reason, Avedis Donabedian, Shan Cretin, Jim Reinertsen, and Brian Jarman. At greater distance, but deeply influential, have been W. Edwards Deming and Joseph Juran. In more recent years, Tom Nolan in particular has become, to my delight and honor, my major mentor and honest critic; it is remarkable to me how much I hear Tom's voice and ideas reflected in my own speeches.

Just as important in shaping my thinking have been my friends and colleagues on the founding board of the Institute for Healthcare Improvement (IHI): Paul Batalden, Dave Gustafson, Jim Schlosser, Vin Sahney, Jim Bakken, Gene Nelson, and Jim Roberts. Successive IHI board members have provided an endless supply of wise guidance and skill-building: Heinz Galli, David Lawrence, Louise Liang, Ellen Gaucher, Judy Miller, Gayle Capozzalo, Bob

Waller, Rick Norling, Martin Harris, Ruby Hearn, Howard Hiatt, Aleta Holub Belletete, David Leach, Gary Mecklenburg, Rudy Pierce, Sister Mary Jean Ryan, Sheila Ryan, Pete Velez, Gail Warden, and Mike Wood. My very career, and the existence of the IHI, can be traced directly to two of these people, both advisers and close friends: Howard Hiatt, who has guided and influenced my work more than any other single individual in my entire life, and Paul Batalden, whose vision and wisdom inform me every day.

Both senior IHI faculty and many colleagues in other countries have added scope to my knowledge, including Laura Adams, Helen Bevan, David Fillingham, Dean Lea, Margareta Palmberg, Wim Schellekens, Richard Smith, and Ross Wilson.

The managers and staff of the IHI provide me with the support and encouragement without which none of my current work, including this book, would be possible. Penny Carver, Carol Haraden, Pat Rutherford, Jonathan Small, Tom Novak, Andrea Kabcenell, and Joanne Healy make up our executive team, and not one of us, least of all me, would have a fraction of our success in hand without the incomparable, wise, optimistic, and patient leadership of Maureen Bisognano—executive vice president and chief operating officer of the IHI and my soul mate, adviser, and comrade in arms.

These speeches, and much of my latter-day writing, have been lovingly and meticulously edited and improved by an IHI publications team whose generosity and competence set a whole new standard for such work: Frank Davidoff, Jane Roessner, and Val Weber. This book is theirs as much as it is mine, except for its defects, which I own.

To my friends Judi and Ken Greenberg—and to their children, Laura, Amy, and Lisa—I owe thanks for the many evenings and long trail hikes over the years, during which they tolerated, with only mild derision, my draft-quality ideas and improved them by thinking with me.

Finally, I thank my family. My children—Ben, Dan, Jessica, and Becca, from whom I have learned what is important and what is not, have played many roles in these speeches. Not always delighted to do so, they appear over and over again as metaphors and examples—soccer players, health care volunteers, wilderness hikers, and always learners—enriching my stories as they enrich my life.

Above all, I thank my wife, Ann, who after all is said and done is by far my best teacher, closest friend, and strongest support. What is not evident to the reader is my debt to Ann and the kids in the hours and hours and days and days of distraction and travel that these speeches represent—precious time borrowed and stolen from the family, testing their patience and drawing on their generosity. They, and I, can only hope that the price we have paid in time lost together will be returned in good measure through whatever impact this book, these speeches, and the work they summarize can have on the future burden of illness for us, for those we love, and for countless others whom we will never know.

Introduction

Frank Davidoff, MD

Don Berwick preaches revolution.

He might not put it quite that way himself—although by his own reckoning he has become increasingly "radicalized" in recent years about the shortcomings of health care. But as the speeches collected in this volume testify, his assessment of the scope and nature of health care's ills and his vision of what health care can and should be are nothing short of revolutionary; nonviolent revolution, to be sure; velvet revolution, perhaps; but revolution nevertheless.

What's he trying to overthrow? His target is a health care system that has evolved primarily to serve the needs and interests of those who work in the system—doctors, nurses, administrators, payers, insurers—rather than the needs and interests of patients. To make matters worse, it's a system (at least in the United States) increasingly caught up in the need to realize investor profits. It's a system characterized by many ills, including ineffectiveness, waste, inefficiency, unnecessary waiting, disorganization, self-interest, harm to patients, disrespect, inequity. In effect, it's a stupid system. Indeed, these speeches make the case that the present state of health care is sufficiently bad that tinkering around the edges is a recipe for failure; only fundamental change—revolution of a kind—will do the job. Berwick's target is definitely not people—neither individual people nor groups or classes of people. On the contrary, his fundamental assumption is that most people who work in the system are smart, dedicated, caring, good people; their frustration as they try to help their scared, hurting patients get better, or get along, in a stupid system is a national, and international, tragedy.

How does Berwick advocate changing the system? All of the speeches in this book reflect three important aspects of Berwick's revolutionary posture. First, he's positive. In his landmark 1989 article, "Continuous Improvement as an Ideal in Health Care,"[1] Berwick turned quality improvement in medicine on its ear by exposing fundamental flaws in the then-current "blame" approach (getting rid of the "bad apples," the outliers at the extremes of the performance curve) and shifting to a process of continuous learning from errors ("every defect is a treasure," moving the entire performance curve upward), as had been happening for years outside of medicine. Ever since then he has been passionate about the need to avoid blame and to maintain hope, even as he lays out the challenge of confronting medical care's ugly realities and doing something effective about them—not an easy balancing act. Second, he recognizes that even at its biological best, medicine is always—*always*—a social act; he understands that changing the system requires fundamental changes in the network of human interactions that drive it—in effect, new and better organization, new and better communication, and new and better system management, at many different levels. Third, he's action oriented; he both expects performance and offers tools for getting it.

What are those tools? Here are some of the most noteworthy:

• *Name the problem.* "Dirty Words and Magic Spells" reflects on the power of accepting reality, of facing up to just how big, how ubiquitous, and how damaging the problems in the health care system really are, and on the power of language—for better or for worse—in defining that reality. (This is not unlike the essential first step in recovery from substance abuse—accepting that you have a problem and that it's gotten out of control.)

- *Build on successes.* We hear about them over and over—for example, the 90 percent reduction in inappropriate use of ICU bed days in one year at York Hospital, and the 50 percent reduction in emergency room waiting time at St. Joseph's Mercy Hospital—in "Why the *Vasa* Sank."

- *Take leaps of faith.* Curing childhood leukemia, long seen as "impossible," happened because some very smart, hardworking people had the courage and imagination to think it wasn't impossible (see "Eagles and Weasels").

- *Look outside medicine.* Medicine can take important lessons from the experiences of General Motors, Canon, General Electric, Alcoa, the airline industry, the Swedish navy, the U.S. Forest Service, and coaching girls soccer, not to mention serious wilderness hiking (see "Run to Space" and "Why the *Vasa* Sank")—and it needs to stop pretending it's unique and has nothing to learn from those outside.

- *Set aims and show constancy of purpose.* Define explicitly where you want to go and when you want to get there, and stick to those goals. These are crucial tasks, and harder to do than they look (see "Buckling Down to Change").

- *Understand systems.* It's not enough to listen well, motivate people, and give them feedback; you also have to understand, explicitly and in detail, how systems work (such as the hierarchy of health care system levels described in "Every Single One"), what it takes to prevent them from collapsing under stress (such as sensemaking through improvisation, virtual role systems, attitude of wisdom, and respectful interaction, described in "Escape Fire"), and how to catalyze the diffusion of innovations within systems (see Berwick's rules in "Sauerkraut, Sobriety, and the Spread of Change")—and leaders can't delegate this understanding.

- *Make action lists.* The speeches included here are full of them. For example, in "Run to Space" we have the following:

1. Reduce waste in all its forms.
2. Study and apply the principle of continuous flow.

3. Reduce demand.

4. Plot measurements related to aims over time.

5. Match capacity to demand.

6. Cooperate.

Such lists belong on the walls of health care organizations, in their daily meetings and talks, and in the consciousness of everyone who works in health care.

- *Never—ever—lose sight of the patient as the central figure*. Making patients and their families truly the force that drives everything else in health care is perhaps the most revolutionary tool of all. Its importance is evident at the system level (see "Every Single One"), but it comes through even more strongly at the personal level (see "Kevin Speaks," "Quality Comes Home," "Escape Fire," and "Dirty Words and Magic Spells").

Why publish these speeches, and why now? Speeches often don't make good reading, for many reasons. First, the rhetoric of speeches is fundamentally different from that of printed text: *Verba volent, scripta manent*—spoken words fly away, written words remain. Because readers can go back over printed text as often as they want, important messages need be stated only once. In contrast, speakers need to underscore key points by repeating them many times and in many ways, which can get in the way in written text. Second, the contexts of the two media are different—the medium really *is* the message. Speeches are real-time social events, and speakers connect directly and immediately with their audiences. Moreover, keynote speeches, such as the ones in this volume, are designed to set the tone for particular meetings and rally the audience to the work at hand. In contrast, print is passive, generic, nonliving; it puts distance, in both time and space, between authors and readers, which can drain the life out of a speech. Third, the audience hears only one speech at a time, so each speech has to stand on its own; publishing all of them together (they're published here almost exactly as they were delivered live) can result in unintended redundancy.

That said, the speeches in this volume have a kind of coherence and energy that translates well to the printed page, which is why several of them have already appeared (slightly edited, to be sure) in print ("Buckling Down to Change" was published in *JAMA* as "Eleven Worthy Aims for Clinical Leadership of Health System Reform"[2]; "Quality Comes Home" was published in the *Annals of Internal Medicine*[3]; "Escape Fire" was published by the Commonwealth Fund[4]; and "Sauerkraut, Sobriety, and the Spread of Change" was published as "Disseminating Innovations in Health Care" in *JAMA*[5]). Besides, people who have heard the speeches live, and others who have heard about them, keep asking for copies. They are telling us that these speeches are helpful to them in the never-ending tasks of setting the tone, rallying people to the cause, and giving people the tools for improvement. Finally, having all the speeches available together makes it possible to examine the trajectory of improvement in medicine over a decade of intense and rapidly developing work, and allows the intrinsic synergy among the speeches to emerge—in fact, not all redundancy is bad, as advertisers and politicians understand very well.

What *don't* the speeches deal with? First, apart from a few passing references (such as to excessive cesarean section rates, inadequate use of risk-reducing medications following myocardial infarction, and inappropriate use of antibiotics), the speeches touch very little on purely clinical, "bedside" issues. This may be because clinical decisions are made between individual patients and their providers, and Berwick is concerned primarily with addressing problems at the systems level. Second, the speeches don't deal head on with a related and difficult problem: the reality of the few people working in health care who aren't up to the job—those who can't judge their limits, others who aren't caring people, still others who are fundamentally disorganized or incompetent, and the very few who are mean-spirited, malicious, or otherwise out of control. The problems created by these people clearly present important challenges for health care, but they're primarily problems with individual people, and although they need serious attention, they very likely require an approach different from, albeit complementary to, system-level interventions. Third, although the intensely positive focus of the speeches is an important part of their effectiveness, they tend to avoid the dark side of improvement work: the barriers to change, the deep sources of resistance to improvement (such as the shame that blossoms in response to the criticism of past performance that is implicit in improvement efforts), the hypertrophied autonomy needs of health care providers, the irrational but locked-in malpractice litigation system, and the perverse financial incentives. Berwick's message is clear in this regard, however: the "blame game" hasn't fixed a stupid system, hence we need to continue avoiding blame, rewarding success, providing hope, and infusing energy.

One of the most important messages of these speeches is that meaningful improvement work depends on collective wisdom—the kind of new meaning, new mental models, and new insights that grow out of true, ongoing dialogue (the word *dialogue* comes from Greek roots: "the meaning flows through"). Much of the power of these speeches comes from Berwick's ability to link ideas spread across wildly different domains, to synthesize ideas that have developed within a huge network of like-minded but widely scattered people, to harness them into a shared vision, and to create a set of working tools for change. By adding large measures of personal energy, passion, and eloquence, Berwick helps listeners, and now readers, to carry the vision, and the tools, around in their heads rather than leave them behind in the lecture hall, or on the page.

Have these speeches changed anything for the better in health care? We don't know now and probably never will, but it's a good bet that they have. Indeed, it's just possible that fifty years from now people will look back and say that Don Berwick's keynote speeches from the 1990s provided one of the sparks that helped set off the revolution in health care. Whether or not that's the future view, these speeches make extraordinarily good reading right now. We know that no one who reads all eleven of them will fail to learn a lot, we doubt that any reader will fail to be entertained, and we challenge any reader to get through all eleven without being deeply moved—perhaps even to the point of personally mounting the improvement barricades.

Notes

1. Berwick, D. M. "Continuous Improvement as an Ideal in Health Care." *New England Journal of Medicine*, 1989, *320*(1), 53–56.

2. Berwick, D. M. "Eleven Worthy Aims for Clinical Leadership of Health System Reform." JAMA, 1994, *272*, 797–802.

3. Berwick, D. M. "Quality Comes Home." *Annals of Internal Medicine*, 1996, *125*, 839–843.

4. Berwick, D. M. "Escape Fire." New York: The Commonwealth Fund, 2002.

5. Berwick, D. M. "Disseminating Innovations in Health Care." JAMA, 2003, *289*, 1969–1975.

Escape Fire

1

Kevin Speaks

Commentary

Susan Edgman-Levitan

Ten years ago, Donald Berwick made an eloquent plea that we should listen to the words of those we serve—our patients and their families. He was right. None of us in health care would have work, do research, teach, or do all of the other things we love without them. Yet *serve* is probably not the right word. *Used* might be a better term for what patients and their families feel about how we care for and interact with them.

The Institute of Medicine has defined eight dimensions of patient-centered care in its report, *Crossing the Quality Chasm*: access to care, respect for patients' preferences, information and education, coordination of care, emotional support, physical comfort, involvement of family and friends, and transition and continuity. These are the most important aspects of care, according to patients and their families.

Has anything changed for patients in this regard since Donald Berwick first told us about the requests of a young patient named Kevin? A few things have improved, including the following:

• Open-access scheduling and improved flow of care in the hospital are providing better access to care.

• Shared decision making is becoming a practical technique for incorporating patients' preferences into the care process. Patients' values should be the principal drivers of their care.

• The Internet has opened up the world of health information and communication to both patients and clinicians. Web sites such as MyGroupHealth.com and PatientSite.com make the medical record, e-mail communication, and other credible health information available. New organizations such as the Center for Information Therapy in Washington, D.C., help clinicians provide evidence-based information to the right patient at the right time via print materials and the Internet.

• Over the last decade, almost fifty hospitals have implemented the model created by Planetree, a pioneer in personalizing, humanizing, and demystifying the health care experience for patients and their families. These hospitals' patients and their families are empowered through information and education and are encouraged to develop "healing partnerships" with caregivers.

• The widespread use of patient-controlled analgesia has perhaps done more to improve patients' physical comfort than any other medical intervention in recent decades.

• Many organizations now open their doors to families and friends in the emergency room, in the recovery room, and in the intensive care unit. Some are even changing their visitor signs to indicate that *providers*, not families, are the visitors in the patient's life.

• The spread of patient and family advisory councils is helping to build a strong foundation for patient- and family-centered care by providing a systematic way to incorporate patients' and families' perspectives into organizational policies and quality improvement priorities.

Sharing clinical pathways and guidelines with patients and their families begins to help with coordination of care, but true coordination is almost impossible to do well in the absence of a real health care *system*. Curiously, health care still has a lot to learn about providing emotional support and preparing people to manage their health problems after they are discharged from the hospital. We don't take advantage of what we know about coping styles, about adult and experiential learning, and about the help that families can provide to support care.

Kevin asked for help with the fundamental issues we all face when we feel vulnerable and need help: "Tell me what you know right away," he asked. "Comfort me, answer me, do not make me wait or waste my time. Try not to frighten me." And most important of all, "Help me, to the very best of your ability, to live and to grow." What is it about the culture of health care that makes it so hard for us to partner with our patients? The things that drive patients crazy also trouble our staff. The system of care for which we are striving will be possible only when we care for the staff, too. They need respect, manageable work, and managers who are accountable and who serve those who are caring for patients. They need time to heal and process difficult emotional encounters. They need information tools to meet patients' needs for information and decision-making support. They need well-designed systems that facilitate superb service, and they deserve reward and recognition for a job well done. Staff need a culture that acknowledges that the best care comes from people working as a team, not as "lone rangers" with sole responsibility for the success or failure of their actions. They desperately need new systems that make the environment safe for them and their patients, one that lets them admit mistakes so that better solutions can be designed for the future.

This new culture requires that the power and autonomy demanded by many who work in health care must go hand in hand with the *responsibility* to meet the needs of patients. A new culture would insist on new models of care that support partnerships with patients, while acknowledging the importance of professional knowledge and expertise. Perhaps someday one's status and pay will even increase commensurately with the healing and compassion one offers, rather than through intellectual intimidation or control over one's peers. Consumers tell us that the term *health care system* is an oxymoron, and we know they are right. We need a real system that supports those who work in it, as well as those who are served by it.

Health care also needs strong leaders who understand the experience of illness and what it is like to be on the front lines day in and day out. We need to recruit and train people who view healing as a vocation, a calling, if you will, at all levels of the system. People like this, working in a system that encourages and rewards their humanity, will instinctively understand how cruel it is to view Kevin's wishes as "unrealistic" and will never again use the excuse, "We're so busy. Doesn't he know he'll have to wait?"

In his book, *A Whole New Life*, Reynolds Price wrote, "It's often said by way of excuse that doctors are insufficiently trained for humane relations. For complex, long-range interactions with damaged creatures, they may well need a kind of training they never receive, but what I wanted and needed badly was the frank exchange of decent concern. When did such a basic transaction between two mammals require postgraduate instruction beyond our mother's breast?" What we all want and need from a new model of care is the same: a system that allows us to connect with our deepest human dignity and respect for one another, care that is relationship-centered at its core, and for it to be no longer *radical* to be kind to one another and especially to sick people. Together we can refuse to check our hearts at the door and find new ways to work together lovingly.

Further Reading

Price, R. *A Whole New Life: An Illness and a Healing*. New York: Atheneum, 1994.

Kevin Speaks

4th Annual National Forum on Quality Improvement in Health Care

Orlando, Florida, December 7, 1992

How far we have come! A mere five or six years ago, the language of quality improvement, if not the ideas themselves, would have met with blank stares in most quarters of American health care. It is not that we did not believe that improvement was necessary, but rather that, simply put, we didn't have a plan.

Now we do—or at least we know what a plan should look like. We know that it must be driven by a constant purpose to be, in the future, something far better than we are today. We know we must change to do this. We know there are principles of customer focus, employee involvement, statistical thinking, project teams and improvement cycles, better reliance on intrinsic motivation, valuing interdependencies, and understanding the system as a whole—principles that are well worth mastering and using in our daily work, and that, properly used, can give us results in cost and quality that, under other sets of management principles, will be out of our reach.

We can now assemble as a group sixteen hundred strong, and many more besides, to explore and build that plan and to shore up our confidence that this is, after all, a plan worth staying with. I look around this room and take renewed energy in the task we have set. We are on a good and sound track, but it is a hard track—hard enough to test our commitment from time to time.

We have to find a constant source of renewed energy. Every now and then, as we feel our sense of safety and commitment tested,

Keynote speech presented at the 4th Annual National Forum on Quality Improvement in Health Care, Orlando, Florida, December 7, 1992.

it is worthwhile for us to touch base with a fundamental question, from which, in the end, the energy to proceed really comes. That question is this: Why improve? What purpose is so important and compelling as to cause us to undertake willingly the dislocation of our systems, our priorities, and our beliefs? To make ourselves uncomfortable?

In the search for will, I always come back to those we serve.

Our purpose comes from those we serve. Continual reconnection to this basic purpose is the only durable source of energy for systemic improvement.

Let Kevin speak. Kevin is fifteen years old. When he was two, a catastrophic problem required the removal of a large portion of his small intestine—the part of the bowel that absorbs nutrition from food. Kevin now has "short gut syndrome"—too little bowel to sustain his growth and health—so for thirteen years he has been fed in part by special intravenous fluids through a plastic tube in a major vein. Nine times in thirteen years that plastic tube has gotten blocked or infected and has therefore had to be surgically replaced. When I spoke with Kevin last, he was in the hospital for yet another replacement of the tube—the tenth—and nobody—not Kevin or me or his surgeon—knew yet if a suitable vein could be found for a new tube. The stakes, obviously, were high.

My medical students had asked me to help them understand the life of a child with chronic illness, so we asked Kevin, the expert (and the customer), to help us. I asked him to write for us on a sheet of paper three things about the care he received that especially pleased him—what he would call "quality"—and three things in which we had failed him—our "defects." This is what he wrote:

Care is best when:

1. They tell you what's going on right away.
2. You get the same answer from everyone.
3. They don't make you scared.

Care is worst when:

1. They keep you waiting.
2. They don't listen to what you say, even when
   sometimes you know better.
3. They do everything twice instead of once.

In the storm of the health care crisis—the variations on "pay or play" or the "Canadian option" or "managed competition"; in the various debates about rationing and protocols and incentive compensation, and even about TQM—it is so easy—frighteningly easy—to forget why we trouble ourselves in the first place. It is so easy— frighteningly easy—to become trapped in the sterile thesis that our institutions must survive simply because they must survive, or that our true, deep purpose is to gain and preserve market share in a vacant terrain of others whose purpose is precisely the same. It is easy to believe that our habits of work are somehow valid and worth defending in isolation from the reason that work exists in the first place.

But the work is not there in the first place. The work is second. In the first place there is Kevin. "Tell me what you know right away," he asks. "Comfort me, answer me, do not make me wait or waste my time. Try not to frighten me," he asks. And unspoken, because he is so frightened, is the most important request of all: "To the very best of your ability, help me live and grow." We are not there to survive. We are there to help Kevin survive.

But we face a problem, because the more we look at Kevin's temperate, respectful, completely understandable requests, the harder they seem to satisfy. That, in fact, is what the medical residents thought when I showed them Kevin's paper. They called Kevin "unrealistic." "We're so busy. Doesn't he know he'll have to wait?" To his request that we give him consistent answers, the residents replied that medicine was too much an art, and at any rate that would require meetings among themselves and with consultants, for which there was no time.

We are trapped. Kevin's requests are reasonable—meeting them is our purpose—yet they are daunting. I asked Kevin to score us on a scale of 0 (meaning never adequate) to 100 (meaning perfect). This is how he scored us:

- They tell you what's going on right away: 35 percent
- You get the same answer from everyone: 30 percent
- They don't make you scared: 40 percent

It is our duty to help Kevin, yet we cannot help him without changing ourselves. There is a strong and inescapable line between the meeting of Kevin's needs, on the one hand, and the methods through which we manage ourselves, on the other. TQM, CQI, systems thinking, improvement—taken in the context of the needs of a frightened fifteen-year-old boy, these are not buzzwords; they are answers to the question, How can we help him better?

Kevin did not put it this way, but he might have: "Be a system," he required of us, "and once you're a system, improve, because I need you to."

Why does the request of a fifteen-year-old boy lead us to such remote corners of self-reflection as systems thinking, process control, and process improvement? It is because Kevin's requests are not requests of parts of us, but requests of the whole. It is inconceivable that any collection of fragments can reliably give this boy what he has every right to expect. Who can make it true that Kevin is not kept waiting, is treated consistently over time and place, and is reassured when and how he needs to be? Who can make it true that Kevin, in our collective hands, is safe—as absolutely safe as he can possibly be? How can we give Kevin the sense he needs that we are all there for him, all together? Whose job is that: The doctor's? The nurse's? The pharmacy's? The school's? The laboratory's? The computer people's? His parents'? His church's? None of those. No list of parts suffices.

Peter Senge describes the fallacies that come from thinking and acting in fragments. His MIT colleague Professor Fred Kofman calls the challenge "recovering the memory of the whole." If we wish to serve Kevin well, we must do it together; if we wish to improve how we serve him, then we must do that together as well. We will think in process terms and improve the processes of our work, or we will let him down. We will be whole, or we will fail.

What is true for Kevin as an individual is even truer for the communities we serve. The waste in health care, its excesses, the gaps in its coverage, and the errors in its services will not yield to conventional approaches. It does not matter all that much how the financing game is changed—under pay-or-play, global budgets, or managed competition. We who make care will still be faced with a choice: either to make that care better, safer, and less costly, or to get by.

They need us to change: the 35 million Americans who lack health insurance need us to change; the one out of four inner-city mothers who lack adequate prenatal care need us to change; the victims of adverse events in one out of every ten hospitalizations; the black citizens of America, whose infant mortality rate is twice that of whites and whose rate of violent death is three times that of whites; the victims of thoroughly preventable deaths from lung cancer, strokes, heart attacks, and premature birth; the elderly whose bed sores can be avoided; the children whose learning disabilities can be avoided; the teenagers who pregnancies can be avoided; the communities whose resources we continue to drain by double-digit rates of increase in health care costs, without any credible defense in the form of scientific proof of effectiveness. They all need us, as much as or more than Kevin does. They need us to be something in the future that we are not today.

When W. Edwards Deming urges us to constancy of purpose, or Joseph Juran instructs us to schedule improvements, or Tom Nolan inquires about what we wish to accomplish, or Peter Senge reminds us of our inescapable systemness, they are doing far more than asking us if we are satisfied with our bottom line. They are not just calling upon us to consider our own adaptive capacities so that we may survive. They are giving us the opportunity to reconnect with the reasons for our being here at all. TQM is worth little or nothing except in the context of fulfilling the aims of our organizations and, through our organizations, the aims of our lives. It is for these reasons that the learning taking place here is so important and, in the end, so thrilling to be a part of.

Kevin said it best when I asked him to tell me more about his simple request that, as he put it, we ask him the same question once, or maybe twice, but not over and over and over again as if we had no memories at all. "It worries me when different people repeat the same question," said Kevin. "Don't you ever talk to each other? Don't you ever meet and agree on what to do? If you don't talk to each other, you might forget me."

Further Reading

Deming, W. E. *Out of the Crisis*. Cambridge: Massachusetts Institute of Technology, Center for Advanced Engineering Study, 1986.

Juran, J. M. *Juran's Quality Control Handbook*. New York: McGraw-Hill, 1988.

Juran, J. M. *Juran on Quality by Design: The New Steps for Planning Quality into Goods and Services*. New York: Free Press, 1992.

Kofman, F., and Senge, P. M. "Communities of Commitment: The Heart of Learning Organizations." In S. Chawla and J. Renesch (eds.), *Learning Organizations: Developing Cultures for Tomorrow's Workplace*. Portland: Productivity Press, 1995.

Senge, P. M. *The Fifth Discipline: The Art and Practice of the Learning Organization*. New York: Doubleday, 1990.

Buckling Down to Change

Commentary

Thomas W. Nolan

The eleven worthy aims proposed by Donald Berwick nearly nine years ago still seem worthy today; is that good or bad? One could argue that it is good: the brilliance of this speech is that it articulates aims that are enduring, measurable, and closely connected to the purpose of health care. The only significant omissions, from today's perspective, are aims associated with patient safety and the health care workforce. In the last nine years, many organizations have experimented with initiatives—ranging from local clinical quality improvement projects to national health care reform—to accomplish the aims that Berwick proposed. Despite these efforts, we cannot celebrate the full achievement of even one of the eleven aims. That is bad. Shall we spend the next nine years trying harder with the same approaches or sulking in hopeless frustration? Perhaps a fresh perspective is needed.

Berwick eloquently entreated the health care community—*as a community*—to accept the challenge of executing major reforms: "However fully these aims are within our reach as a system, not one of these aims is within the grasp of *any individual or group acting alone.*" One of the conclusions that can be reached about the last nine years is that these aims are not within the grasp of *the health care system acting alone*. The system is more complex and the problems more intractable than almost anybody predicted. Creative solutions have been limited in part by the domination of biomedical knowledge and the exclusion of the broader range of knowledge that is required to optimize health care systems for the benefit of patients. For example, the complex problem of waiting times cannot be solved without clinicians interacting with those trained in queuing methods and system flow. Typically these persons are engineers, operations researchers, and statisticians. Initially it will be difficult to build these relationships. The "outsiders" will appear naive, overconfident, or uninformed; they will be quick to make analogies to other industries before learning the complexities of health care, and slow to provide specifics. The health care "insiders" will be just as quick to assume that those who don't have biomedical knowledge or health care experience cannot help. With some persistence and good will, however, these different perspectives can be reconciled by agreeing on a common purpose for collaboration: to achieve improved results for patients.

Some courageous and creative members of the health care community have begun to engage similarly courageous and creative outsiders in experiments at the fringes of the current system to create some radically different solutions; many more will need to do so in the future. Examples of such fringe projects might include the following:

- Collaboration with persons experienced in computer network design, multinational product distribution, or automobile traffic flow to develop and execute innovative structures for the flow of patients, supplies, and information in hospitals or other acute care settings.

- Collaboration with persons responsible for managing and assuring the reliability of airline maintenance or air traffic control (systems that require technical knowledge as well as professional judgment to balance risks and costs) to design a safer health care system.

- Association with reliability engineers and experts in supply chain management to design reliable supply chains of clinical knowledge across the continuum of the health care system so that the system delivers a near-perfect match of care with existing scientific evidence and the patient's values.

- Engagement of marketing specialists and a group of representatives of an organization (for example, a company of more than three thousand employees) to work with guidance but not interference from doctors, nurses, and other clinicians to design care that is customized to the health care needs of the people in that organization. That care system would be optimized to attract those people to participate in their own care whether they are sick or well.

- Alliance with executives of multinational companies to understand how they ensure that their employees balance local needs with a global perspective; use of the alliance to build the capability to investigate outside the borders of the United States to learn, for example, how other developed countries are able to deliver babies safely with cesarean section rates that are less than half of our rates, or to learn how to identify waste in our system by observing how some developing countries with per capita health care spending at a fraction of ours are able to provide reasonable levels of health care.

Readers of this speech will be impressed with the extent of the ambition of the eleven aims and with the coherent description of the purpose of health care reform. Ambitious aims must be accompanied, however, by methods equal to the task of accomplishing them. When W. Edwards Deming, one of the developers of the modern philosophy and methods associated with quality and quality improvement, was asked by a student how a complex organization should approach the improvement of quality, he answered, "There is no substitute for knowledge." The health care community would do well to heed Deming's advice and add to its already prodigious biomedical knowledge the knowledge necessary to optimize the health care delivery system. Designing a hospital system so that patients flow smoothly and appropriately from the community to the emergency department to various levels of intensity of care is a daunting task, but so too is the task of designing the hardware and the logic of message flow that allows the global Internet to function. These designers have knowledge that would help in the design of the logic of hospital flow.

Clinicians and health care executives must be curious about the type of system knowledge used in other sectors of society if they desire to develop the methods that will be necessary to accomplish Berwick's eleven aims. For each of the aims, the reader might ponder what industry or country has accomplished related aims or solved equally complex problems. This reflection will open many fruitful paths for collaboration, learning, and progress on the eleven aims.

Buckling Down to Change

5th Annual National Forum on Quality Improvement in Health Care

Orlando, Florida, December 6, 1993

Perhaps like me you look back over the years to certain key moments when some event entered your life and changed your mind forever. Before the event, you saw things one way; afterward, irrevocably, you saw things differently. These are moments of change.

Let me tell you of two such moments for me.

One moment was on a day in 1985 when I first met Guy Cohen, who was then Director of Reliability, Quality, and Safety at NASA. In 1985, NASA still enjoyed a reputation from the days of Gemini and Apollo for its innovative, world-class approach to quality. In an effort to help me understand the NASA quality culture, Guy told me a story that I have never forgotten.

The Titan rocket was a mainstay of the space program in the era before manned flight. In 1958, a Titan rocket failed and the cause was traced to a problem in the liquid oxygen tanks. Liquid oxygen was drawn from these tanks, ten feet in diameter, through an extremely high-pressure pump, and to prevent the pump from undergoing "cavitation," which is caused by the kind of swirling you see as your bathtub drains, metal baffles were placed at the bottom of the tank. Unfortunately, as it turned out, these baffles acted as partial dams to prevent the full use of the liquid oxygen in the tank and, as a result, the fuel ran out a bit early and the rocket missed its target.

Keynote speech given at the 5th Annual National Forum on Quality Improvement in Health Care, Orlando, Florida, December 6, 1993. A version of this speech was published subsequently as "Eleven Worthy Aims for Clinical Leadership of Health System Reform," JAMA, 1994, 272(10), 797–802. Copyright © 1994 American Medical Association.

The solution was to trim some metal from the baffles—a tricky job that required removing a cover from the top of the fuel tank and then lowering a man in a parachute harness with a separate breathing supply on a rope with block and tackle into a tank filled with nitrogen. The man's job was to unbolt the baffle, trim it, and bolt it back into place. The trimming made two bolts on the baffle unnecessary, so the man was to bring these now-unnecessary bolts with him when he was hauled up and out of the tank. A loose bolt in the tank would surely be drawn into the high-pressure pump and cause the rocket to explode upon launch.

The quality team from Martin Marietta carried out this hazardous and expensive job on the launch pad, and with the worker safely recovered, they refixed the top hatch and refilled the tank with protective nitrogen gas. Minutes later, however, a problem appeared. Two bolts were to have been brought to the surface, but the worker had only one. He seemed to remember that the bolt had in fact never been there at all—left out at manufacturing, he thought—but the risk was too great, so the team again opened the tank, removed the hatch cover, and peered with lights and binoculars into the cavernous tank. No bolt was there, they all agreed, and, reassured, they closed the hatch again. Launch was the next morning.

But Gerry Gonsolves couldn't sleep that night. Gerry was a junior quality control officer—a "kid," says Guy Cohen, who was worried. He had been sent to the assembly plant in Denver to act as the "missile chaperone" for the next Titan to be sent to Florida for launch. In the wee hours of the morning, he crawled from his bed and drove to a storage plant where there happened to be a spare, identical twin of the liquid oxygen tank he had inspected on the launch pad. On hands and knees, with a spare bolt and some transparent tape, Gerry crawled in and out of the tank, seeing if just possibly he could fix the loose bolt into a location that was invisible from the open hatch. He found two such locations.

At 2:00 A.M. he awoke his boss, Guy Cohen, at home to tell him of the hazard. "We could have missed the bolt," Gerry told Guy. "We might have screwed up."

With the authority to do so, Guy scrubbed the launch. At 8:00 the next morning, instead of watching a rocket lift off, the team was reassembled on the launch pad. Again they lowered the man into the tank. It took him thirty seconds to find the loose bolt, precisely in one of the two spots that Gerry Gonsolves had identified the night before.

"What did NASA do?" I asked Guy, expecting a story of investigation, censure, and new inspections—the history of quality failures in health care.

"We gold-plated the bolt," said Guy, "and made a tie clip out of it for Gerry. The quality control director presented the award on the day that Titan was finally launched—and hit its target. It was more important to reward, not censure, to make certain that accurate information would flow freely and not be covered up."

I thought of my own world of malpractice suits, quality assurance investigations, performance reviews, and incentive compensation, and then I thought of the world Guy Cohen was describing with that story—a world of openness, involvement, celebration, and dedication to excellence—and I forever changed my mind.

The second story is about me. I was an intern in adult medicine, caring one night in 1973 for a dying woman with severe diabetic ketoacidosis. The acid levels in her blood had built up so high that her heartbeat was weakened and, in a vicious cycle, her body tissues, deprived of their usual blood supply, generated even more acid, which weakened her heartbeat further. We—the team of doctors and nurses—had struggled at her bedside all day long, trying every trick we knew to break that cycle, but her blood pressure kept falling and her death was imminent.

Now there was only me. It was after midnight and the other doctors were asleep. I was on duty and stood by her bedside helpless as she drifted further into shock. I thought of sleeping, but I did not.

Then, somewhere in the back of my mind, a connection was made. Several months before I had attended a lecture on a different kind of acidosis than this woman's, requiring a different kind of treatment, and the lecturer had introduced a surprise: for some forms of acidosis, intravenous methylene blue might theoretically provide some short-term relief.

I decided to try it. The biochemistry made sense, and a short-term fix—a few minutes of better acid balance—might allow her heart to clear some acid and begin to reverse the vicious cycle.

I do not recall this woman's name, nor do I have any idea where she is today or whether she is alive or dead. What I do recall is the tracing on the blood pressure monitor, minute by minute, first slowing its fall and then rising perceptibly, minute by minute, and then her spontaneous breathing returning, and then her first voluntary movements, and then, thirty minutes later, her opening her eyes and looking at me. Three days later, the attending doctor who had expected to sign this woman's death certificate signed her discharge papers instead.

Why did we do this? Why did Gerry Gonsolves wake up in the middle of the night to try again, once more, to find a bolt that he and his entire team had decided, only hours before, was not there? Why did I, an intern at the bedside, tired and drained, think back almost involuntarily to a little piece of information, perhaps irrelevant, and try again, try still, to do what up until that moment had been impossible? Why do we care so much? We care because we feel it is our duty to do so. It is our craft. But this sense of duty does not come from outside; it arises from within. No reward can create this caring. It can be driven out of us, but it cannot be driven into us.

This sense of duty is driven by aims, by knowing what one is trying to accomplish. We achieve focus of effort through focus of aim. Gerry awoke, and I did not sleep, because of the clarity of our purpose and the intensity with which we held it in mind.

Now, in health care, among the people at this Forum, we have made the needed preparations for change. Our preparations are sufficient. We have studied enough. We have reviewed our cultures enough. We have spent the time we needed, enough time, in training and planning and filling our kit with new and useful tools and methods. We know *how*. Now, we must remember *why*.

It seems to me that we could now accomplish a great deal indeed if we could focus our newfound skills on exactly that set of achievements that we will agree to use as the yardstick of our success. If we can pick our aims clearly, we can now buckle down and reach for them. I propose eleven aims for our work over the next two years— eleven needed results that, if achieved, would represent the first solid steps toward the systemic change that is worthy of the name *health care reform*. They are as follows:

AIM 1: *Reduce the use of inappropriate surgery, hospital admissions, and diagnostic tests.*

Important initial targets include management of stage 1 and stage 2 breast cancer,[1–3] prostatectomy,[4] carotid endarterectomy,[5] coronary artery bypass surgery,[6] treatment of low-back pain,[7] hysterectomy,[8] endoscopy,[9] blood transfusion,[10] chest roentgenograms,[11] and pre-natal ultrasound.[12]

A procedure is inappropriate in a particular patient if there is no scientific basis on which to predict benefit. The relationship between variation in practice and inappropriate care is far from straightforward; high-use areas are not necessarily areas of high inappropriateness.[13–15] Research consistently shows, however, that inappropriate surgery,[13–18] admissions,[19] and testing[20,21] are common; for a group of carefully studied surgical procedures, the rate of inappropriate use ranges between 20 and 70 percent.[14] Thanks to a decade of development by scholars at RAND and elsewhere, simple and reliable procedures exist for assessing the appropriateness of care, and these procedures can be adapted for use by physicians in community settings.[22] Specific, targeted efforts to involve clinicians in peer-comparison studies, education, and collaborative guideline development often lead to substantial declines in procedure rates, with a consequent reduction in both costs and hazards to patients.[23]

Those who regulate, measure, or purchase health care understandably tend to treat this problem of inappropriateness from their own outside perspective—hence the current infatuation with protocols, guidelines, algorithms, and critical paths. The trend is worrisome. A guideline enforced from outside may lead to more predictable care, but it cannot lead to the continual improvement of care. The outsider can judge care, but only the insider can improve it.

The commitment to improving the match between scientific knowledge and actual practice, the commitment to "appropriateness," must come from the professionals—nurses, physicians, and managers—whose actions constitute the care. To improve appropriateness, we must begin with a clearheaded understanding that in our hands unnecessary care does exist; it is our well-meaning inappropriateness, it is pervasive, and physician by physician, organization by organization, we can reduce it without guilt, censure, or severe external controls.

AIM 2: *Improve health status through reduction in underlying root causes of illness.*

The underlying root causes of illness include smoking,[24–29] handgun violence,[30–33] preventable injuries in children,[34–36] and alcohol[37] and cocaine abuse.[38] The causes of the majority of both deaths and years of potential life lost in the United States are preventable.[39,40] McGinnis and Foege have recently offered a brilliant reclassification of "actual causes of death" in the United States, showing that tobacco, diet, and activity patterns as well as toxic agents, firearms, sexual behavior, motor vehicles, and illicit use of drugs account collectively for 50 percent of all deaths each year in the United States.[41] Unintentional injuries, suicide, and homicide account for 30 percent of all years of potential life lost under the age of sixty-five.[42]

In their own office-based practices, clinicians have substantial opportunities to affect some of the behavioral causes of illness. Skilled counseling by physicians can reduce smoking, high-risk sexual activities, and some forms of unintentional injury. With simple questionnaires, clinicians can detect alcohol abuse and depression in earlier and less hazardous stages.[43] In large measure, however, knowledge about the social, behavioral, and environmental causes of disease frustrates physicians. How can we, trained as we are in curative care and palliative care after the fact, ever really reach the sources of the illnesses we treat? Is it, after all, our job to do so?

Strong social currents suggest that it may be. Social support for public health and prevention is resurging,[43] reflected in governmental budgets, community-wide health status improvement efforts, and an emphasis on primary care in many health system reform proposals. Of course, so far the signals are still mixed, as every physician knows. No one pays yet for a physician to become a leader in community-wide prevention of automobile accidents, in smoking cessation programs, or in handgun control. A specialist paid thousands of dollars for the terminal care of a cirrhotic patient is paid little or nothing for community work to prevent alcohol abuse. A hospital, such as the Magic Valley Medical Center in Twin Falls, Idaho, that successfully reduces head injuries in children by leading community-wide bicycle safety efforts[44] still takes a significant negative hit on its bottom line because it loses emergency department revenues as a result. No one yet totals and adjusts the economics to encourage more and more preventive activity in the nation.

Yet the duty remains. Even though health care financing currently works against it, a commitment to improvement requires that clinicians carry their work effort to the sources of disease. Physicians strongly influence community attitudes toward appropriate health investments; it is therefore important for physicians not just to countenance prevention but also to lead it.

AIM 3: *Reduce cesarean section rates to below 10 percent without compromise in maternal or fetal outcomes.*

Cesarean section rates in the United States have risen from 5 percent to 26 percent over two decades.[45] Rates well below 10 percent have been maintained in some other developed nations[46] (and as low as 1.3 percent in certain practice settings[47]) without any demonstrated compromise in maternal and fetal outcomes.

In industries other than health care, dramatic improvements have sometimes been motivated by the setting of "stretch goals"— goals that are so demanding that they challenge prevailing assumptions and automatically require reconsideration of the system as a whole. A stretch goal makes the need for fundamental change clear, because it is absolutely unattainable within the existing work process. The cesarean section rate is a candidate for stretch goals. Returning safely to the U.S. rates of the mid-1970s (well below 10 percent) will require fundamental system changes.[48,49] However, we know that it can be done, because others have done it.

AIM 4: *Reduce the use of unwanted and ineffective medical procedures at the end of life.*

Only a minority of patients, families, and clinicians support prolonged use of life-sustaining procedures and dramatic interventions in the terminal stages of illness,[50,51] yet substantial use of these procedures continues.[52] In human terms, using unwanted procedures in terminal illness is a form of assault. In economic terms, it is waste. Several techniques, including advance directives[53] and involvement of patients and families in decision making,[54,55] have been shown to reduce inappropriate care at the end of life, leading to both lower cost and more humane care from the patients' point of view.

It is, of course, hard to know in advance that this month or this week is the last month or week of a patient's life. That is, in fact, one of the main reasons why this particular improvement challenge rests squarely on the shoulders of clinicians. It requires our highest skills to help patients and families balance the factors of uncertainty, dignity, risk, and reward involved in using medical procedures appropriately as life ends. We must begin by recognizing that today the appropriate balance is badly missing.

AIM 5: *Adopt simplified formularies and streamline pharmaceutical use.*

This aim applies especially to antibiotics and to drug prescriptions for the elderly and chronically ill. Medication prescribing errors,[56,57] overuse of antibiotics[58] (especially broad-spectrum antibiotics), and inappropriate polypharmacy in the elderly and chronically ill[59,60] are well documented. Simplified formularies and educational interventions among clinicians[61,62] lead to safer and less expensive prescribing practices. In addition, simplifying the processes by which we order, prepare, and deliver medications should reduce error rates. One hospital system has reported recurrent annual savings of nearly $1 million by using simple ways to ensure the timely administration of correct perioperative prophylactic antibiotics.[63]

This aim is given special urgency by the early warnings we now have about new strains of organisms resistant to multiple antibiotics.[58,64] The wisest possible use of antibiotics may help to slow the emergence of resistance.

AIM 6: *Increase the frequency with which patients participate in decision making about medical interventions.*

A growing amount of experimental literature documents the payoff from helping patients consider explicitly their own values and goals in the context of difficult treatment decisions. "Activated patients" encouraged to ask questions and to participate with their physicians in reaching the best plan of diagnosis and therapy often achieve better outcomes at lower cost than patients in more passive modes.[65,66] This approach does not work for all patients, but it does for many, and it challenges clinicians and organizations to develop new skills and processes for interacting with patients.

The financial gains are substantial. Prostatectomy candidates who help decide between medical and surgical treatment choose surgery as much as 50 percent less often than those for whom the physician alone makes the choice.[67] Diabetic patients who are coached by nonphysicians to ask questions when they see their physicians have lower glycohemoglobin levels and higher functional status than those who are not coached.[68] Chronically ill adults who develop simple self-efficacy skills show subsequent medical utilization patterns 50 percent lower than matched controls.[69]

AIM 7: *Decrease uninformative waiting of all types.*

In health care, experienced physicians sometimes use "watchful waiting" to gain information and to allow natural healing to proceed. This is a sound strategy, often preferable to aggressive clinical intervention. However, a large proportion of the waiting that occurs in health care is not of this informative type; it adds no value for either the caregiver or the consumer of care. In fact, rapid access and high responsiveness are among the major quality characteristics desired by the beneficiaries of health care.[70] Modern companies outside the health care system devote a great deal of attention to reducing such waits throughout the chain of production of a product or service. They aim for continuous flow; they reject batching in favor of more agile, streamlined manufacturing processes.[71] Constructing feasible wait-free processes under constrained resources demands high levels of process redesign and invention, but it leads to markedly improved quality at much lower cost.

In the buffeted health care economy, with wholesale budget cuts now common, more waiting may appear to be inevitable as a device for rationing scarce services.[72] The vocabulary of limitation becomes an acceptable and common form of adjustment to resource constraints. It is precisely at such times, however, that waiting must be unmasked as the thief it really is. Queues often add cost and rob opportunities as more and more time and energy pour into managing waiting lists and enforcing rules of access. Patients who fear that they will be denied care are often thereby induced to demand it, if only to test for their own security. The anger of someone denied access wastes time in apology, defense, and repair.

Organizations and physicians who find new ways to minimize delays, produce continuous flows, and decrease waiting, even while resources are more and more limited, will also find themselves developing innovations that please patients more while stressing and demoralizing caregivers less. The precondition to success is that caregivers must suspend their disbelief long enough to join whole-heartedly in trying out ways to reduce waiting under conditions of severe resource constraint. Testing different ways to reduce or eliminate waiting may be fruitful in appointment-scheduling systems, referral patterns, gatekeeping habits, and administrative barriers to utilization. Several group practices have already had exciting successes with open-access primary care systems in which the patient, not the system, chooses the exact appointment date and time. A hospital committed to reducing waits might refuse to delay admissions pending prospective certification by payers, but guarantee repayment of any charges from admissions that are decertified after the fact.

AIM 8: *Reduce inventory levels.*

Other industries have dramatically reduced their inventory levels through the use of "just-in-time" process flows, improved supplier management, and process simplification.[70] By comparison, health care organizations maintain high inventory levels and tend to underuse capital equipment.[73-75]

At first glance, inventory alone may seem to explain so little of the cost structure of health care that its reduction would not be a significant gain; but look again. Inventory reduction to 10 percent of historical levels, which other industries have achieved, saves money in obvious ways by freeing capital, decreasing storage space, and simplifying record keeping, for example. In less obvious and even more important ways, however, a system that can minimize its own inventory levels may well be fundamentally less expensive to manage and more adaptive to changing needs. If we must store a thousand copies of a form because we cannot be sure that one will be delivered when we need it, we must either throw away or use up our stocks when we need a new version. A system that could deliver forms to us reliably, exactly when needed, would by its nature have to be in close communication with us and thereby better able to understand our needs and more likely to change quickly when necessary.

What do physicians have to do with so administrative a matter as inventory levels? A great deal. By standardizing their requests for materials and services, and by taking the time to explain their needs carefully to their suppliers, physicians can help smooth the flow of supplies through their own system of work and, as a happy by-product, reduce both waits and waste.

Take, for example, the inventory of hip prostheses in an orthopedic unit. Imagine that eight surgeons in a group demand that a dozen different prostheses be available. To have sufficient backup stocks of prostheses on hand, the purchasing office must maintain twelve processes for ordering and storage—one per prosthesis type. The purchasing office must manage multiple outside supplier contracts, with attendant legal, accounting, and clerical costs. The operating room central supply service must maintain a complex storage and retrieval system so that Dr. Jones always receives his proper tray and Dr. Smith hers. If there are ten technicians in central supply, each of whom must be trained in the preferred setup for each of the twelve prostheses, then 120 prosthesis-technician dyads exist. Even if each dyad functions perfectly, with 99 percent probability, the probability of systemic perfection (with all 120 dyads correct) is approximately 0.99^{120}, or 0.30. (This is the joint probability of 120 independent events all occurring together if each has a 99 percent chance of occurring.)

Compare this system with one in which eight surgeons agree, through conversation, research, and compromise, to stock only three prostheses instead of twelve. Inventory decreases, as do the costs of accounting, contracting, storage, tracing, and staff training. Higher-volume purchases from a single supplier will earn price breaks for the hospital. Instead of 120 prosthesis-technician dyads to maintain, there are now only 30, and the probability that the dyads will function correctly is 0.99^{30} or 0.74, a 250 percent improvement. The reduced complexity also creates the opportunity to learn quickly the outcomes of having chosen the particular prostheses (because in a single orthopedic unit it is easier to study three than to study twelve), thus setting the stage for scientifically informed changes in the future selection of prostheses. By exactly this change (reducing the number of hip prostheses in use), one hospital system has saved almost $1 million per year while improving functional status outcomes for total hip replacement patients.[76]

The key point is that physicians and nurses themselves must understand and drive this movement toward reduced complexity and lower inventory. Simplification will make the most sense not when it's thrust on them, but when it's sought and planned with and by them. What applies to hip prostheses applies equally well to many types of durable medical equipment, consumable supplies, examining room stocks and designs, paper forms, and procedure-manual specifications. In a group of eight pediatricians, how many types of standing orders should there be for support staff to follow to prepare a toddler for examination? The common answer is eight. The correct answer, if we truly value both quality and efficiency, is one.

AIM 9: *Record only useful information only once.*

Let us define *useful* as "likely to be used by someone, sometime." By this measure, medical records, administrative habits, and regulatory history require extraordinary levels of "useless"— wasteful, duplicative, and unused—record keeping, both clinical and administrative.[77–79] Decreasing duplicate data entry and ceasing the recording of information that is never used would both reduce costs and improve care. To accomplish this goal requires rational changes in regulation and, even more important, changes in outmoded habits and information management systems. Some changes may be outside the jurisdiction of physicians and nurses, but many useless habits are preserved by administrative fiat or by internal governance committees on forms and medical records. In all arenas, nursing and physician leaders should insist on rational parsimony and should discard recording practices honored by time but not by logic. How often do we record vital signs and why? Why do separate sections of the medical record contain virtually the same information? How many times do patients have to tell us their telephone numbers? Do we record quantitative information in daunting tables or in informative graphs? Simply substituting graphs for tables and lists of numbers in our medical records would be a big step forward.

As they seek simplified and less wasteful record keeping, clinicians should question the ever-present, intimidating trump card of "medical-legal requirements." Some of these requirements are indeed worth worrying about, but many are myths—durable but wrong. In some cases, the risks of nonrecording may be well justified by savings in both time and money. An automated medical record may provide a partial solution, but it will be little help if it merely stores magnetically the waste formerly stored on paper.

AIM 10: *Reduce the total supply of high-technology medical and surgical care and consolidate high-technology services into regional and community-wide centers.*

The largest single determinant of the rate of high-technology care and invasive procedures is the level of local supply of those services.[19,80–82] For many high-technology practices, reduction in the total supply is an effective and safe way to reduce costs and limit adverse medically induced outcomes.

When this reduction is achieved through consolidation, we can expect outcomes to improve. Encouraging data suggest a positive relationship between "volume" and "outcomes," especially with regard to high-technology services, although the full profile of this relationship is not yet known.[83–88] Duplication of services results in higher costs, higher usage rates, and inefficient use of capital. Some benefits from regional consolidation have been documented for care of very low birth weight infants[89] and for adult cardiac surgery.[90] Most metropolitan areas in the United States should reduce the number of centers engaging in cardiac surgery, high-risk obstetrics, neonatal intensive care, organ transplantation, tertiary cancer care, high-level trauma care, and high-technology imaging.

This is not an easy change for physicians to accept. Some physicians in high-technology specialties will lose income and job opportunities as a result. For-profit, entrepreneurial providers of medical imaging, renal dialysis, and outpatient surgery, for example, may find their business opportunities constrained. It will be necessary for other physicians, who see the benefits of consolidation of services, to insist on sensible regionalization nonetheless, even at the risk of internal professional conflicts. Courage in medicine now includes the courage not to demand the highest level of technology "right here, on site," but to seek instead the more challenging forms of integrated, interinstitutional relationship that in the long run achieve more for less.

AIM 11: *Reduce the racial gap in health status, beginning with infant mortality and low birth weight.*

Extreme differences remain in infant morbidity and mortality rates for minorities and low-income populations compared with whites of higher economic status in the United States.[91,92] The causes are multifactorial,[93] so multiple system improvements will be required to reduce the gap.

Perinatal outcomes are only the tip of the iceberg of social inequity in the health status of Americans.[94–96] Not only are black infants 240 percent more likely than whites to die in the perinatal period, but they also face a far more uncertain future if they live. A black male born today in the United States has the following excess risks of death compared with a white male: 150 percent for heart disease, 190 percent for stroke, 280 percent for renal disease, 340 percent for human immunodeficiency virus–related death, and 680 percent for homicide.[97] Life expectancy for a black male at birth today is eight years less than for a white male; for a black female, it is six years less.[96]

These discrepancies are not only offensive, they are also insupportable. Any national or regional changes worth calling "reform" in health care, any agenda worth calling "improvement," must intend explicitly to reduce this injustice.

The problem of infant mortality and low birth weight is a fine place to begin. The potential gains are large, the measurement systems to support tests of change are feasible, and the implications for cost, as well as for outcomes, are favorable. Results will come only from highly integrated, collaborative action at the community level, and solutions will vary based on local conditions. Medical leadership of this community-wide activity is essential, not only to ensure that health care organizations allocate their own resources where they will do the most good, but also to stimulate the conscience of the public and to convene organizations and individuals in pursuit of common goals. The increasing investment in severe competition in many local medical markets will prevent such collaborative action unless clinical leaders, driven by their ethical duty, insist on it.

These eleven aims define an action plan for clinicians who wish to lead effective change in U.S. health care. Any hospital, integrated system, or community making substantial gains in even half of these areas would be easily distinguishable in cost, outcome, and satisfaction. Costs would decrease dramatically as a result of decreases in inappropriate and unwanted care, simplified pharmaceutical use, less supply-driven use of medical procedures, reduced record keeping, and less complex inventory. Health status indicators would reveal decreases in preventable morbidity and mortality, more individualized patient care decisions, and fewer complications from drugs, invasive tests, and surgical procedures. If community-wide action were taken, the gaps between white and minority health status would begin to close. Patients would report shorter waiting times, more respectful dialogues with their health care providers, and less duplicative and disorganized care. In short, such a system of care would be better, cheaper, and incidentally more satisfying to work within.

A good case exists for other aims as well, but the real point is for physicians to get started and to engage in improving specific dimensions of care as quickly as we can. Physicians who wish to help lead systemic change toward aims such as these will likely have to cultivate new personal skills. To accomplish each of these improvements, the heroic image of individualist physicians each doing the best he or she can and each bearing full and personal responsibility for the care of the patient cannot possibly suffice. These aims reflect the performance of systems of interdependency, not of individuals acting alone. They will be accomplished by those who provide health care, or they will not be accomplished at all. Physicians who wish to help must learn more than how to heal patients; they must also learn how to heal systems.

Healing systems will require skills not customarily taught in medical training. Progressive medical education in the future should help physicians, nurses, and administrators to participate fully in changing the systems in which they do their work. Relevant skills include the following: the ability to understand the health care system as a whole, not merely one's own profession; the ability to gather and interpret data on outcomes of care; the ability to work effectively across disciplinary boundaries and, when needed, to participate in formal improvement teams; the ability to trust generally in the motives and intelligence of people in different professional roles, of different genders, and with different life experiences; the skill and willingness to test new approaches to work instead of clinging to the status quo as the safest option; and the ability to interpret the underlying needs of patients and others who depend on physicians, so the definition of "needed improvements" will be placed firmly in the hands of those who are served by the health care system.[98]

What a wonderful achievement it would be if each of us could return to this Annual Forum in 1994 and then 1995 and then 1996 and thereafter with reports in hand, documenting wise measurements of gains made at least in these eleven areas of performance. Suppose we could celebrate, in one year or two or three, not just that we have learned statistical thinking, or practiced meeting skills, or understood the dynamics of systems or PDCA cycles, but that, as a result of our work, fewer and fewer black babies are being born with low birth weight; that fewer and fewer unnecessary carotid endarterectomies are being done; that head injuries in children and smoking in adults have fallen by 50 percent; that only 9 percent of all births are now by cesarean section; that our metropolitan areas have cut in half the number of centers performing organ transplants and coronary surgery and, as a result, reduced the complications of those procedures by a third; and that our patients wait measurably less and are involved measurably more in the choices that affect their lives in prostate surgery, chemotherapy, and the management of coronary disease.

What if, in short, we could report to each other next year, and year by year afterward, that we have made changes that produce exactly what we are after: much better outcomes, much better caring, much more justice, and much lower cost—all at the same time.

It will not happen in Washington. It will not happen in your state capital. It will not happen because someone buys right, or pays right, or judges right. It will not happen because of consumer choice, or managed competition, or single payers, or global budgets. These rules and conditions only set the stage—they are not at all the play.

It will happen if and only if we, the people in this room, decide to make it happen. And if we use the methods we now know to accomplish what we really want. And if we do it together, because, to whatever degree these aims are within our reach as a system, not one of them is within the grasp of any individual or group act-ing alone.

We are at the bedside again, but this time we are together. The others have left. Now it is just us, and the patient—our sys-tem. The duty remains. Shall we sleep?

Notes

1. Farrow, D. C., Hunt, W. C., and Samet, J. M. "Geographic Varia-tion in the Treatment of Localized Breast Cancer." *New England Journal of Medicine*, 1992, *326*, 1097–1101.

2. Lazovich, D., White, E., Thomas, D. B., and Moe, R. E. "Under-utilization of Breast-Conserving Surgery and Radiation Therapy Among Women with Stage I or II Breast Cancer." *JAMA*, 1991, *266*, 3433–3438.

3. Nattinger, A. B., Gottlieb, M. S., Veun, J., Yahnke, D., and Good-win, J. S. "Geographic Variation in the Use of Breast-Conserving Treatment for Breast Cancer." *New England Journal of Medicine*, 1992, *326*, 1102–1107.

4. Wennberg, J. E., Mulley, A. G., Jr., Hanley, D., and others. "An Assessment of Prostatectomy for Benign Urinary Tract Infection: Geographic Variations and the Evaluation of Medical Care Out-comes." *JAMA*, 1988, *259*, 3027–3030.

5. Winslow, C. M., Solomon, D. H., Chassin, M. R., and others. "The Appropriateness of Carotid Endarterectomy." *New England Journal of Medicine*, 1988, *318*, 721–727.

6. Winslow, C. M., Kosecoff, J. B., Chassin, M., Kanouse, D. E., and Brook, R. H. "The Appropriateness of Performing Coronary Artery Bypass Surgery." *JAMA*, 1988, *260*, 505–509.

7. Deyo, R. A. "Fads in the Treatment of Low Back Pain." *New Eng-land Journal of Medicine*, 1991, *325*, 1039–1040.

8. Bernstein, S. J., McGlynn, E. A., Siu, A. L., and others. "The Appropriateness of Hysterectomy: A Comparison of Care in Seven Health Plans." *JAMA*, 1993, *269*, 2398–2402.

9. Kahn, K. L., Kosecoff, J., Chassin, M., Solomon, D. H., and Brook, R. H. "The Use and Misuse of Upper Gastrointestinal Endoscopy." *Annals of Internal Medicine*, 1988, *109*, 664–670.

10. Soumerai, S. B., Salem-Schatz, S., Avorn, J., Casteris, C. S., Ross-Degnin, D., and Popovsky, M. A. "A Controlled Trial of Educational Outreach to Improve Blood Transfusion Practice." *JAMA*, 1993, *270*, 961–966.

11. Crain, E. F., Bulas, D., Bijur, P. E., and Goldman, H. S. "Chest X-rays Are Often Unnecessary in Febrile Neonates." *Pediatrics*, 1991, *88*, 821–824.

12. Ewigman, B. G., Crane, J. P., Frigoletto, F. D., and others. "Effect of Prenatal Ultrasound Screening on Perinatal Outcome." *New England Journal of Medicine*, 1993, *329*, 821–827.

13. Chassin, M. R., Kosecoff, J., Park, R. E., and others. "Does Inappropriate Use Explain Geographic Variations in the Use of Health Care Services? A Study of Three Procedures." *JAMA*, 1987, *258*, 2533–2537.

14. Brook, R. H., Park, R. E., Chassin, M. R., Solomon, D. H., Keeney, J., and Kosecoff, J. "Predicting the Appropriate Use of Carotid Endarterectomy, Upper Gastrointestinal Endoscopy, and Coronary Angiography." *New England Journal of Medicine*, 1990, *323*, 1173–1177.

15. Leape, L. L., Park, R. E., Solomon, D. H., Chassin, M. R., Kosecoff, J., and Brook, R. H. "Does Inappropriate Use Explain Small-Area Variations in the Use of Health Care Services?" *JAMA*, 1990, *263*, 669–672.

16. Franks, P., Clancy, C. M., and Nutting, P. A. "Gatekeeping Revisited: Protecting Patients from Overtreatment. *New England Journal of Medicine*, 1992, *327*, 424–429.

17. Friedman, B., and Elixhauser, A. "Increased Use of an Expensive, Elective Procedure: Total Hip Replacements in the 1980s." *Medical Care*, 1993, *31*, 581–599.

18. Einstadter, D., Kent, D. L., Fihn, S. D., and Deyo, R. A. "Variation in the Rate of Cervical Spine Surgery in Washington State." *Medical Care*, 1993, *31*, 711–718.

19. Wennberg, J. E., Freeman, J. L., and Culp, W. J. "Are Hospital Services Rationed in New Haven or Overutilized in Boston?" *Lancet*, 1987, *1*, 1185–1188.

20. Griner, P. F., and Glaser, R. J. "Misuse of Laboratory Tests and Diagnostic Procedures." *New England Journal of Medicine*, 1982, *307*, 1336–1339.

21. Axt-Adarn, P., van der Wouden, J. C., and van der Does, E. "Influencing Behavior of Physicians Ordering Laboratory Tests: A Literature Study." *Medical Care*, 1993, *31*, 784–794.

22. Kosecoff, J., Chassin, M. R., Fink, A., and others. "Obtaining Clinical Data on the Appropriateness of Medical Care in Community Practice." *JAMA*, 1987, *258*, 2538–2542.

23. Weingarten, S., Agocs, L., Tankel, N., and others. "Reducing Lengths of Stay for Patients Hospitalized with Chest Pain Using Medical Practice Guidelines and Opinion Leaders." *American Journal of Cardiology*, 1993, *71*, 259–262.

24. Adams, M. M., Brogan, D. J., Kendrick, J. S., and others. "Smoking, Pregnancy, and Source of Prenatal Care: Results from the Pregnancy Risk Assessment Monitoring System." *Obstetrics & Gynecology*, 1992, *80*, 738–744.

25. Chilmonczyk, B. A., Salmun, L. M., Megathlin, K. N., and others. "Association Between Exposure to Environmental Tobacco Smoke and Exacerbations of Asthma in Children." *New England Journal of Medicine*, 1993, *328*, 1665–1669.

26. Higgins, M. W., Enright, P. L., Kronmal, R. A., Schenker, M. B., Anton-Culver, H., and Lyles, M., for the Cardiovascular Health Study Research Group. "Smoking and Lung Function in Elderly Men and Women: The Cardiovascular Health Study." *JAMA*, 1993, *269*, 2741–2748.

27. Janerich, D. T., Thompson, W. D., Varela, L. R., and others. "Lung Cancer and Exposure to Tobacco Smoke in the Household." *New England Journal of Medicine*, 1990, *323*, 632–636.

28. Schoendorf, K. C., and Kiely, J. L. "Relationship of Sudden Infant Death Syndrome to Maternal Smoking During and After Pregnancy." *Pediatrics*, 1992, *90*, 905–908.

29. Seidman, D. S., Ever-Hadani, P., Gale, R., and others. "Effect of Maternal Smoking and Age on Congenital Anomalies." *Obstetrics & Gynecology*, 1990, *76*, 1046–1050.

30. Kellermann, A. L., Rivara, F. P., Sornes, G., and others. "Suicide in the Home in Relation to Gun Ownership." *New England Journal of Medicine*, 1992, *327*, 467–472.

31. Kellermann, A. L., Rivara, F. P., Rushforth, N. B., and others. "Gun Ownership as a Risk Factor for Homicide in the Home." *New England Journal of Medicine*, 1993, *329*, 1084–1091.

32. Koop, C. E., and Lundberg, G. D. "Violence in America: A Public Health Emergency—Time to Bite the Bullet Back." *JAMA*, 1992, *267*, 3075–3076. Corrections: *JAMA*, 1992, *268*, 3074; *JAMA*, 1994, *271*, 1404.

33. Loftin, C., McDowall, D., Wiersema, B., and Cottey, T. J. "Effects of Restrictive Licensing of Handguns on Homicide and Suicide in the District of Columbia." *New England Journal of Medicine*, 1991, *325*, 1615–1620.

34. Centers for Disease Control. "Fatal Injuries to Children: United States, 1986." *Morbidity and Mortality Weekly Report*, 1990, *39*, 442–445.

35. Chorba, T. L., and Klein, T. M. "Increases in Crash Involvement and Fatalities Among Motor Vehicle Occupants Younger Than Five Years Old." *Pediatrics*, 1993, *91*, 897–901.

36. Thompson, R. S., Thompson, D. C., Rivara, F. P., and Salazar, A. A. "Cost-Effectiveness Analysis of Bicycle Helmet Subsidies in a Defined Population." *Pediatrics*, 1993, *91*, 902–907.

37. Centers for Disease Control. "Alcohol-Related Traffic Fatalities During Holidays: United States, 1989." *Morbidity and Mortality Weekly Report*, 1989, *38*, 861–863.

38. Phibbs, C. S., Bateman, D. A., and Schwartz, R. M. "The Neonatal Costs of Maternal Cocaine Use." *JAMA*, 1991, *266*, 1521–1526.

39. Fries, J. F., Koop, C. E., Beadle, C. E., and others. "Reducing Health Care Costs by Reducing the Need and Demand for Medical Services." *New England Journal of Medicine*, 1993, *329*, 321–325.

40. U.S. Department of Health and Human Services, U.S. Public Health Service. *Healthy People 2000: National Health Promotion and Disease Prevention Objectives*. Washington, D.C.: U.S. Department of Health and Human Services, 1990.

41. McGinnis, J. M., and Foege, W. H. "Actual Causes of Death in the United States." *JAMA*, 1993, *270*, 2207–2212.

42. Centers for Disease Control and Prevention. "Years of Potential Life Lost Before Age Sixty-Five: United States, 1990 and 1991." *Morbidity and Mortality Weekly Report*, 1993, *42*, 251–253.

43 U.S. Preventive Services Task Force. *Guide to Clinical Preventive Services: An Assessment of the Effectiveness of 169 Interventions*. Baltimore: Williams & Wilkins, 1989.

44. Roessner, J. "The Healthiest Place in America." *Quality Connection*, 1993, *2*, 10–11.

45. Bottoms, S. F., Rosen, M. G., and Sokol, R. J. "The Increase in the Cesarean Birth Rate." *New England Journal of Medicine*, 1980, *302*, 559–563.

46. Centers for Disease Control and Prevention. "Rates of Cesarean Delivery: United States, 1991." *Morbidity and Mortality Weekly Report*, 1993, *42*, 285–289.

47. Rockenschaub, A. "Technology-Free Obstetrics at the Semmelweis Clinic." *Lancet*, 1990, *335*, 977–978.

48. Lopez-Zeno, J. A., Peaceman, A. M., Adashek, J. A., and Socol, M. L. "A Controlled Trial of a Program for the Active Management of Labor." *New England Journal of Medicine*, 1992, *326*, 450–454.

49. Flamm, B. L., Newman, L. A., Thomas, S. J., and others. "Vaginal Birth After Cesarean Delivery: Results of a Five-Year Multicenter Collaborative Study." *Obstetrics and Gynecology*, 1990, *76*, 750–754.

50. Garrett, J. M., Harris, R. P., Norburn, J. K., and others. "Life-Sustaining Treatments During Terminal Illness: Who Wants What?" *Journal of General Internal Medicine*, 1993, *8*, 361–368.

51. Gray, W. A., Capone, R. J., and Most, A. S. "Unsuccessful Emergency Medical Resuscitation: Are Continued Efforts in the Emergency Department Justified?" *New England Journal of Medicine*, 1991, *325*, 1393–1398.

52. Lubitz, J. D., and Riley, G. F. "Trends in Medicare Payments in the Last Year of Life." *New England Journal of Medicine*, 1993, *328*, 1092–1096.

53. Emanuel, L. L., Barry, M. J., Stoeckle, J. D., Ettelson, L. M., and Emanuel, E. J. "Advance Directives for Medical Care: A Case for Greater Use." *New England Journal of Medicine*, 1991, *324*, 889–895.

54. Townsend, J., Frank, A. O., Fremont, D., and others. "Terminal Cancer Care and Patients' Preference for Place of Death: A Prospective Study." *British Medical Journal*, 1990, *301*, 415–417.

55. Smedira, N. G., Evans, B., Grais, L., and others. "Withholding and Withdrawal of Life Support from the Critically Ill." *New England Journal of Medicine*, 1990, *322*, 309–315.

56. German, P. S., and Burton, L. C. "Medication and the Elderly: Issues of Prescription and Use." *Journal of Aging and Health*, 1989, *1*, 5.

57. Lipton, H. L., and Bird, J. A. "Drug Utilization Review in Ambulatory Settings: State of the Science and Directions for Outcomes Research." *Medical Care*, 1993, *31*, 1069–1082.

58. Cohen, M. L. "Epidemiology of Drug Resistance: Implications for a Post-Antimicrobial Era." *Science*, 1992, *257*, 1050–1055.

59. Bernstein, L. R., Folkman, S., and Lazarus, R. S. "Characteristics of the Use and Misuse of Medications by an Elderly, Ambulatory Population." *Medical Care*, 1989, *27*, 654–663.

60. Lesar, T. S., Briceland, L. L., Delcoure, K., Parmalee, J. C., Masta-Gornic, V., and Pohl, H. "Medication Prescribing Errors in a Teaching Hospital." *JAMA*, 1990, *263*, 2329–2334.

61. Avorn, J., and Soumerai, S. B. "Improving Drug-Therapy Decisions Through Educational Outreach: A Randomized Controlled Trial of Academically Based 'Detailing.'" *New England Journal of Medicine*, 1983, *308*, 1457–1463.

62. Kimberlin, C. L., Bernardo, D. H., Pendergast, J. F., and McKenzie, L. C. "Effects of an Education Program for Community Pharmacists on Detecting Drug-Related Problems in Elderly Patients." *Medical Care*, 1993, *31*, 451–468.

63. Classen, D. C., Evans, S., Pestotnik, S. L., Horn, S. D., Menlove, R. L., and Burke, J. P. "The Timing of Prophylactic Administration of Antibiotics and the Risk of Surgical Wound Infection." *New England Journal of Medicine*, 1992, *326*, 281–286.

64. Neu, H. C. "The Crisis in Antibiotic Resistance." *Science*, 1992, *257*, 1064–1073.

65. Wennberg, J. E. "Improving the Decision-Making Process." *Health Affairs* (Millwood), 1988, *7*, 99–106.

66. Greenfield, S., Kaplan, S. H., and Ware, J. E., Jr. "Expanding Patient Involvement in Care: Effects on Patient Outcomes." *Annals of Internal Medicine*, 1985, *102*, 520–528.

67. Kasper, J. F., Mulley, A. G., and Wennberg, J. E. "Developing Shared Decision-Making Programs to Improve Quality of Health Care." *Quality Review Bulletin*, 1992, *18*, 183–190.

68. Greenfield, S., Kaplan, S., Ware, J. E., and others. "Patient Participation in Medical Care: Effects on Blood Sugar Control and Quality of Life in Diabetes." *Journal of General Internal Medicine*, 1988, *3*, 448–457.

69. Sobel, D. S. "Mind Matters, Money Matters: The Cost-Effectiveness of Clinical Behavioral Medicine." In *Mental Medicine Update: Special Report*. Los Altos, Calif.: Center for Health Sciences, 1993.

70. Ware, J. E., and Snyder, M. K. "Dimensions of Patient Attitudes Regarding Doctors and Medical Care Services." *Medical Care*, 1975, *13*, 669–682.

71. Womack, J. P., Jones, D. T., and Roos, D. *The Machine That Changed the World*. New York: HarperCollins, 1991.

72. Grumet, G. W. "Health Care Rationing Through Inconvenience: The Third Party's Secret Weapon." *New England Journal of Medicine*, 1989, *321*, 607–611.

73. Redelmeier, D. A., and Fuchs, V. R. "Hospital Expenditures in the United States and Canada." *New England Journal of Medicine*, 1993, *328*, 772–778.

74. Thorpe, K. E. "Inside the Black Box of Administrative Costs." *Health Affairs* (Millwood), 1992, *11*, 41–55.

75. Woolhandler, S., and Himmelstein, D. U. "The Deteriorating Administrative Efficiency of the U.S. Health Care System." *New England Journal of Medicine*, 1991, *324*, 1253–1258.

76. Weed, M., written communication, February 1994.

77. Woolhandler, S., Himmelstein, D. U., and Lewontin, J. P. "Administrative Costs in U.S. Hospitals." *New England Journal of Medicine*, 1993, *329*, 400–403.

78. Institute of Medicine. *The Computer-Based Patient Record: An Essential Technology for Health Care*. Washington, D.C.: National Academies Press, 1991.

79. Weed, L. L. "Medical Records That Guide and Teach." *New England Journal of Medicine*, 1968, *278*, 593–600, 652–657.

80. Greenfield, S., Nelson, E. C., Zubkoff, M., and others. "Variations in Resource Utilization Among Medical Specialties and Systems of Care: Results from the Medical Outcomes Study." *JAMA*, 1992, *267*, 1624–1630.

81. Schroeder, S. A., and Sandy, L. G. "Specialty Distribution of U.S. Physicians: The Invisible Driver of Health Care Costs." *New England Journal of Medicine*, 1993, *328*, 961–963.

82. Welch, W. P., Miller, M. E., Welch, H. G., Fisher, E. S., and Wennberg, J. E. "Geographic Variation in Expenditures for Physicians' Services in the United States." *New England Journal of Medicine*, 1993, *328*, 621–627.

83. Every, N. R., Larson, E. B., Litwin, P. E., and others. "The Association Between On-site Cardiac Catheterization Facilities and the Use of Coronary Angiography After Acute Myocardial Infarction. *New England Journal of Medicine*, 1993, *329*, 546–551.

84. Farber, B. F., Kaiser, D. L., and Wenzel, R. P. "Relation Between Surgical Volume and Incidence of Postoperative Wound Infection." *New England Journal of Medicine*, 1981, *305*, 200–204.

85. Flood, A. B., Scott, W. R., and Ewy, W. "Does Practice Make Perfect? The Relation Between Hospital Volume and Outcomes for Selected Diagnostic Categories." *Medical Care*, 1984, *22*, 98–114.

86. Laffel, G. L., Barnett, A. I., Finkelstein, S., and Kaye, M. P. "The Relation Between Experience and Outcome in Heart Transplantation." *New England Journal of Medicine*, 1992, *327*, 1220–1225.

87. Luft, H. S., Bunker, J. P., and Enthoven, A. C. "Should Operations Be Regionalized? The Empirical Relation Between Surgical Volume and Mortality." *New England Journal of Medicine*, 1979, *301*, 1364–1369.

88. Luft, H. S., Hunt, S. S., and Maerki, S. C. "The Volume-Outcome Relationship: Practice-Makes-Perfect or Selective Referral Patterns?" *Health Services Research*, 1987, *22*, 158–182.

89. Boyle, M. H., Torrance, G. W., Sinclair, J. C., and Horwood, S. P. "Economic Evaluation of Neonatal Intensive Care of Very-Low-Birth-Weight Infants." *New England Journal of Medicine*, 1983, *308*, 1330–1337.

90. Showstack, J. A., Rosenfeld, K. E., Garnick, D. W., Luft, H. S., Schaffarzick, R. W., and Fowles, J. "Association of Volume with Outcome of Coronary Artery Bypass Graft Surgery: Scheduled vs. Nonscheduled Operations." *JAMA*, 1987, *257*, 785–789.

91. Centers for Disease Control. "Low Birth Weight: United States, 1975–1987." *Morbidity and Mortality Weekly Report*, 1990, *39*, 148–151.

92. Wegman, M. E. "Annual Summary of Vital Statistics." *Pediatrics*, 1993, *92*, 743–754.

93. Kempe, A., Wise, P. H., Barkan, S. E., and others. "Clinical Determinants of the Racial Disparity in Very Low Birth Weight." *New England Journal of Medicine*, 1992, *327*, 969–973.

94. Guralnik, J. M., Land, K. C., Blazer, D., Fillenbaum, G. G., and Branch, L. G. "Educational Status and Active Life Expectancy Among Older Blacks and Whites." *New England Journal of Medicine*, 1993, *329*, 110–116.

95. Sommer, A., Tielsch, J. M., Katz, J., and others. "Racial Differences in Cause-Specific Prevalence of Blindness in East Baltimore." *New England Journal of Medicine*, 1991, *325*, 1412–1417.

96. Pappas, G., Queen, S., Hadden, W., and Fisher, G. "The Increasing Disparity in Mortality Between Sociodemographic Groups in the United States, 1960 and 1986." *New England Journal of Medicine*, 1993, *329*, 103–109.

97. Centers for Disease Control. "Years of Potential Life Lost Before Age Sixty-Five, by Race, Hispanic Origin, and Sex: United States, 1986–1988." *Morbidity and Mortality Weekly Report*, 1992, *41*(suppl. SS6), 18–19.

98. Berwick, D. M., Enthoven, A., and Bunker, J. P. "Quality Management in the NHS: The Doctor's Role." *British Medical Journal*, 1992, *304*, 235–239, 304–308.

3

Quality Comes Home

Commentary

Brian Jarman

When I read Donald Berwick's speech my first reaction was,
"Don's father needed a good general practitioner (GP), as good
a GP as he was himself." He needed someone who was conver-
sant with his medical condition and his social circumstances,
preferably over a period of years, whom he trusted and who had
the authority to act for him with clarity and decisiveness. My
second reaction, after a little thought, was, "The good GP needs
to be working in a good, caring health care system"—one whose
purpose is healing and caring for patients. Not a health care
industry, but a system that is designed purposefully to emphasize
the healing of and caring for patients, not the profits to be made
from that activity. A good GP would have been able, with the
help of the family, to integrate the patient's care by visiting the
patient regularly (particularly important if the relatives live far
away) and bringing to bear his particular knowledge of that particular patient.

I worked as a GP within the United Kingdom's National
Health Service (NHS) for twenty-eight years. For the last fourteen years I spent half of my time as a professor of primary health
care. The more difficult but more worthwhile job was that of providing good continuing care for patients and their families who

were registered with me, on my "panel." Luckily I worked within a system in which health care was not looked on as an industry in which maximizing profits was of vital importance. The national health care system can itself have problems if there is too heavy-handed or, even worse, incompetent organization by a central government. However, within the NHS I always had the feeling that the system was humane and reasonably patient-centered. I never had to bill a patient and could concentrate my energies on healing and caring for them. I would have liked more resources at times, but on the whole in my practice we managed pretty well and I felt that the patients received good care. We didn't have to deal with "five different evaluation forms . . . , with five different recommendations, for five separate fees."

A large, centralized—some would say paternalistic—health care system such as the NHS can, because of its centralized nature, be one in which it is difficult for health care professionals to work locally in an innovative way, with the government "breathing down your neck." The culture tends to discourage thinking of new ideas—for instance, developing measurement methods designed to improve care—and more generally doing the things that the Institute for Healthcare Improvement is so good at fostering. For this reason I believe that the NHS must change to a system in which provider hospitals, primary care groups, and trusts (which are responsible for commissioning care from providers for their registered patients) can act innovatively on their own, with only quality control and resource allocation being the province of the central organization.

When reading Berwick's speech I thought of a story that an American friend told me in the late 1990s of a colleague who made many millions of dollars by arranging for a reorganization of health care systems that were similar, I imagine, to the ones Berwick describes. At the time, I wondered how much the patients involved benefited from this reorganization. If health care is treated as an industry, as though it were making cans of beans or whatever, then competition between hospitals could, and probably already does, easily lead to the situation where access to the information needed to provide excellent care could be restricted in order to give particular hospitals a competitive advantage. Similarly, any health care system in which the profit motive is dominant and that is based primarily on commercial insurance will inevitably lead to greater cost to those individuals who have the greatest health care problems and are least able to afford health care—thus leading to a proportion of the population not having health care coverage. In my opinion, in a civilized society the purpose should not be to maximize the profits of insurance companies. As Berwick reminds us, "The enemy is disease. The competition that matters is against disease, not one another. The purpose is healing."

It cannot be beyond the wit of man to create a system of health care that provides primary care for the entire population (which might represent about 6 percent of the total costs, excluding medications prescribed) and that provides all secondary health care (for which there is meaningful evidence of its value). For some conditions, such as acute appendicitis, there would be no need for detailed studies regarding the evidence base, but for other conditions, such as infertility, there would need to be a decision, perhaps at the state level, as to what care should be covered. Doing this would involve bringing in non–health care professionals for advice in order to learn from the experience of others and use the enormous amount of information that already exists. But first there must be a willingness to "just get started."

Quality Comes Home

6th Annual National Forum on Quality Improvement in Health Care

San Diego, California, December 4, 1994

Few people know that I am an avid Star Trek buff. Even fewer care. But those among you who share this addiction with me— even those among you who will not admit it—know that special moment when Captain Jean-Luc Picard, with Klingon warbirds hurtling toward him, with shields at half strength and decreasing, with the reserves of trilithium crystals dangerously low, and with the fate of the galaxy hanging by a thread, warms up the warp drive, raises his index finger, and gives the command, "Engage." There is no moment in Shakespeare more satisfying.

That's the theme of this speech: "Engage." It's time. And we are ready. And the Klingons approach. If I could accomplish one thing in the next hour, it would be to convince you that the means for acceleration are at hand, among us. Our problem is no longer to achieve success. It is to define success as "what really matters."

A one-word summary of the state of mind of the health care system last year—1993—might have been *anxious*. We were in suspension, holding our breath, waiting for health care reform's shoe to drop.

Not this year. Now the word is not *anxious*. We are well beyond anxious. A better word is *confused*. *Chaos* would do too. The shuffling is awesome: mergers and acquisitions, downsizing and layoffs, budget cuts and price slashing, integrating and competing. Physi-

Keynote speech presented at the 6th Annual National Forum on Quality Improvement in Health Care, San Diego, California, December 4, 1994. A version of this speech was published subsequently as "Quality Comes Home," *Annals of Internal Medicine,* 1996, *125*(10), 839–843.

cian groups that eighteen months ago were scheming to keep managed care out of town are now hiring consultants to help them decide next week with whom to make an exclusive contract before they get shut out of the action.

The Institute for Healthcare Improvement (IHI) recently offered a course for about forty people on a topic of current concern. Eleven CEOs were in the room. One took an urgent phone call to find out that he had just been fired. That same week I spent time with a hospital director who was in the process of laying off 10 percent of his employees. He cried. An ear, nose, and throat surgeon in private practice in upstate New York pulled me aside at a meeting and said, "I want to improve, but my overhead is killing me. I don't think I have time. I've never been so scared in my life."

I've never been so scared in my life. Those words seem melodramatic, but they are not too far off the mark. Scared, and confused. There is an underlying rumble in the health care world, even among the apparently confident dealmakers and the apparently successful executives who end up at the top of the merger, that—really, deeply, way down inside, and usually unspoken—they have not got a clue about what to do. It might shock some of you to know the names of executives who this year, trusting me, in the quiet of their office or a local lounge have said, "This is crazy. We are all running around, and no one knows what to do. All we know is that doing nothing seems unacceptable. We're all afraid of being left out. But left out," they ask, "of what?"

Never before in the recent history of health care in North America has common sense been so uncommon. I sometimes feel as if I am watching an anthill on which some passing hoof has trodden. So much scurrying, but to what end? What?

Dr. W. Edwards Deming made constancy of purpose the first and most crucial of his famous Fourteen Points for Top Leaders. Today, constancy seems farthest from our minds.

It is at times like this that returning home may be most crucial. To touch base. To remember. To center ourselves once again.

Quality came close to home for me as an issue this year. I was reminded, with unwelcome vividness, of the kind of constancy we really need—of what, behind the chaos of mergers and acquisitions, downsizing and layoffs, budget cuts and price slashing, integrating and competing, is worth the trouble. It involved my father.

My father is a retired physician in rural Connecticut. For forty-two years he provided care as a general practitioner to a population of farmers, laborers, and their families in the tiny town in which I grew up. Now, at age eighty-four, he no longer gives care, he receives it.

I do not know what he thinks of health care reform. By the time the national issue became popular, my father was unable mentally to comprehend the debate. He could not define or even recognize managed care, alliances, integrated systems, AHCPR guidelines, or PHOs. I don't think he knows what TQM stands for, and he would probably define *reengineering* as changing the person who drives a freight train.

Of course he does know quality. He is the guy who got up in the middle of the night to drive out to the Balec farm because Jimmy had a high fever. I would become half awake at the sound of his car starting in the driveway, but I would not know why until the next morning, when I heard about Jimmy's fever or Mr. Bernstein's heart attack or the awful car accident at the drawbridge. I heard my father speak rudely to patients sometimes, but I never saw him unconcerned. And when I attended my thirtieth high school reunion in the town this year, I was still Dr. Berwick's boy. People could not wait to remind me of the time my father delivered their baby—or them—or sewed up a wound or answered a tough question. Not a great doctor, perhaps, but a good one. He was always there, they said. You could count on him.

My father retired ten years ago, and not long afterward began developing symptoms of Parkinson's disease and mild dementia from small, multiple strokes. He remained alert and took joy in his grandchildren, but became progressively weaker, until one day this past June he fell and broke his hip. I want to tell you the story.

He fell at home. He tottered once too often up the three eight-inch steps to his bedroom and fell forward on his head and hip, bruising one and breaking the other. His housekeeper found him and called the ambulance.

One of my brothers, who lives an hour from our father's home, rushed to the local hospital to meet him in the emergency room. There he asked for my father. He was told, in error, that our father was not there. Panicked phone calls followed as my brother searched anxiously for our father, until finally someone told him that our father was there after all and was about to be wheeled to the operating room.

After surgery, my father lay sedated on a special mattress containing sections that alternately inflated and deflated. Within a week he had a deep pressure ulcer on his right heel. It was painful and interrupted his early ambulation therapy. He became restricted to a wheelchair for most of the day and gradually refused to walk at all.

Unable to return home, my father needed to go to a rehabilitation facility, and my brothers and I searched hard for the best one. We interviewed visiting nurses, physical therapists, and local doctors—and the signals pointed to a facility twenty miles from his home. It was the best place of its kind around.

I visited him there on the morning after his admission. He was lying stuporous in the bed, on his back, with his ulcerated heel pressing into the sheets. His mouth was hanging open and his eyes were rolled back into his head. I asked the nurse for an explanation. "We sedated him," she said. "He was combative. He hit a staff member." For ten years my father has had severe Parkinson's disease, and for most of that time he has been unable to extend his own arm voluntarily, much less throw a roundhouse punch. My father had undoubtedly been angry, yes. But a punch—no. I demanded that the sedation be stopped.

Not that it mattered much. For reasons that never became clear, his Parkinson's medication, meticulously adjusted for two years by his physician at home, was stopped summarily when he was admitted to the rehabilitation facility. This resulted in a two-week siege of spasm and much decreased mobility.

Not that that mattered much, either, however. By then the pressure sore on his right heel had opened again, causing pain that prevented him from walking or even spending much time in a wheelchair.

Not that it mattered, because when my brothers and I asked that our father be placed in a wheelchair whenever possible, the weekend shift of nurses told us that no wheelchairs could be found. They asked that we bring in his rickety old wheelchair from home. They eventually did find a wheelchair, but it was missing the footrest plate that would have protected his injured heel from bruising.

My father spent six weeks in the rehabilitation facility and then gave up, as did the staff. He returned home to a hospital bed and around-the-clock housekeeper coverage. Two weeks after he got home—almost entirely bedridden and almost certainly never to walk again—a wheelchair finally came: the latest model, with postural supports, custom back rests, and hand controls he can never use. We never asked for it; the home care company simply ordered it. It's beautiful. The price: $6,000. It sits proudly and nearly unused in the corner of his bedroom.

It is very hard to convey to you the special sense of helplessness I feel as a participant in this. One year ago I stood before sixteen hundred National Forum attendees in Orlando to set an agenda for improvement. I proposed eleven aims for clinical leadership of change that really would matter. Aim 5 called for more appropriate use of pharmaceutical agents, especially with the elderly. But I find my own father heavily oversedated with sleeping pills he does not need and dramatically undermedicated with the anti-Parkinson's agents he does need. Aim 4 called for the appropriate use of technology, especially in the last stages of life; but I find an excessively complex and nearly useless $6,000 wheelchair freighted to my father's home, whereas a far simpler one could not be found during the week in which it would have made a real difference. Aim 7 asked that we decrease the amount of time spent waiting, but my own brother sits uninformed and confused for four hours in the waiting area of an emergency department.

Aim 2 involved prevention, including prevention of injuries, but my own father, seemingly inevitably, falls at home, and inevitably acquires a debilitating and totally preventable pressure ulcer that irreversibly interrupts his rehabilitation.

I feel helpless. So does he.

So many stories in health care are now layered over with the jargon and catechisms of our search for some better way. My father would never have asked for "integrated delivery," but only to be passed gently and securely from the hands of one caring person to the other. He wanted no "guidelines" or "critical paths," but instead reliability and promises that he could count on. He is less interested in "cost containment" than in the simpler aim that he not be harmed with waste or avoidable pain. He would not ask for "access"; he would ask instead that we be there when he needs us. And now, he needs us. We did not do well enough. He did not get what he has earned and, in my opinion, has a right to expect.

Yet behind this story, and beyond the anger, I also feel a sense of possibility. In the course of my work I am privileged to see good news as well as bad. In place after place, I see throughout the health care systems of the United States and Canada an ever-increasing collection of glowing successes that rivet my attention. Let me show you some examples.

My father was oversedated; it did not need to be that way. At Intermountain Health Care's Latter-Day Saints (LDS) Hospital in Salt Lake City, Utah, the director of critical care medicine, Dr. Terry Clemmer, the nurse manager of that unit, Vicki Jensen Spuhler, and their colleagues have worked for two years on safe sedation, substituting a class of older, safer, and less costly agents for new, expensive drugs whose use had become prevalent. Total savings for Intermountain Health Care has been $209,000, with far safer levels of sedation for patients in the intensive care unit.

Dr. Ken Peterson and his colleagues in pediatrics at the Alaska Native Medical Center in Anchorage have been working on improvements in the sedation of children undergoing computed tomography. As a result of their efforts, the rate at which procedures had to be rescheduled because of ineffective sedation decreased from 40 percent in May 1993 to less than 1 percent in September 1994.

Improvement in medication has been a goal of John Burke and the infectious disease group at LDS Hospital since the mid-1980s. Through the group's work during the past seven years, antibiotic costs are down almost $60,000 per year and have decreased from 25 percent to 13 percent of the pharmacy budget. Duration of therapy has been shortened, and outcomes from infections have improved.

My father was never successfully rehabilitated from his hip fracture because the rehabilitation system failed him at crucial points. It didn't need to be that way. Working with a team in his center, Dr. Bill Nugent, chief of cardiothoracic surgery at Dartmouth-Hitchcock Medical Center in Lebanon, New Hampshire, has been able to reduce both median postoperative length of hospital stay and mortality rates after heart surgery by carefully preparing patients for postoperative care and rehabilitation.

Drs. Michael Morris and Peter Mandt, orthopedic surgeons at Virginia Mason Medical Center's Sports Medicine Clinic in Seattle, Washington, have led a total redesign of their repairs of anterior cruciate ligament tears. Between 1993 and 1994 they reduced actual costs of care by almost $1,500 per patient, from $4,501 to $3,031, while sustaining a clinical success rate of 96 percent and a return to work at one year rate of 100 percent.

My father's rehabilitation was permanently stalled by a pressure ulcer on his foot. It did not need to be that way. Prevention of pressure ulcers has been the subject of a major guideline by the Agency for Health Care Policy and Research. This guideline was studied and used by a team at LDS Hospital under the leadership of Carol Ashton. The team celebrated a decrease in pressure ulcer rates on a medicine service—from 24 percent during July to December 1992, to 2.7 percent during January to June 1993. For the patients at highest risk, the rate of ulcers in that period fell from 37 percent to less than 10 percent.

For my brother, the emergency department was a place to wait, questions unanswered, misinformed, anxious. It did not need to be that way. Carolyn Jackson and Dr. Andrew Greene at Bethany Hospital in Chicago, Illinois, converted their emergency care for adults with asthma into the first step in a carefully integrated sequence of patient and family education, evaluation, and support. Between 1992 and 1994, returns of asthma patients to the emergency department decreased from 11.6 patients per month to 2.3 patients per month; rehospitalization rates were cut by 60 percent and adults' inpatient length of stay for asthma decreased by 30 percent.

In Dr. Terry Clemmer's intensive care unit, careful work on improving communications with families over three years has increased the rate at which families are oriented within twenty-four hours of their relative's admission to the intensive care unit from 30 percent to 98 percent.

Through systematic improvement efforts, committed persons have achieved stunning success in areas ripe for clinical breakthrough. I suggested last year that we can, if we wish, safely reduce the rate of cesarean section in the United States from the current 23 percent to below 10 percent. Many health care professionals have doubted that this is possible, citing threats of malpractice suits and patient expectations. But Drs. Robert DeMott and Herbert Sandmire from Green Bay, Wisconsin, reduced the community-wide rate of cesarean sections from 16.3 percent in 1986 to 10.4 percent in 1993. Dr. Charles Guise, from the obstetrics services at the U.S. Air Force Academy Hospital, reports that the rate of this procedure decreased from 17 percent in 1989 to 6 percent in 1993; during the same interval, the rate of vaginal birth after cesarean section increased from 30 percent to 85 percent. In both cases, outcomes for mothers and babies stayed the same or improved.

Improvement is within our reach. Not marginal improvement, but fundamental, breakthrough-level changes that are better for patients, better for families, better for clinicians, and better for payers.

Yet my father now lies in bed in his small Connecticut town and will never walk again.

What will it take?

I asked that question of Carol Ashton, the LDS Hospital nurse whose leadership has saved many unnamed patients the pain and debility of the bedsores that wrecked my father's chances for recovery. "What was it," I asked Carol, "that helped you do this? Why did you succeed?" She named four factors and asked me to tell you about them.

Factor one, she said, *was the ability to involve people*—"front-line people," she calls them—*in the decision to change*. For Carol Ashton, improvement and involvement are not separable. The former depends on the latter.

Factor two was science—she calls it "research-based clinical practice"—*the ability to find and communicate sound reasons for change*— a plausible approach, backed by plausible evidence. Nurses were trained, she found, to rub reddened spots. But that, it turns out, increases ulcer formation. It irritates irritated tissues, accelerating the breakdown of skin. Stopping the practice involved not a protocol or edict but an explanation, offered by credible advisers in a trustworthy setting.

Factor three was a willingness to "just get started," and to trust the capacity of people to make mid-course corrections in improvement processes that would never have been begun if they had to be perfect at the start. Carol Ashton and her colleagues trusted themselves and their ability to "learn as you go."

Factor four, according to Carol, *was support from the organization.* LDS Hospital treated improvement of pressure ulcer prevention not as after-hours work but as work itself. The team was given the time, the data, the analytic resources, and the license to make changes. The money was spent on staff education, team meeting time, data collection resources, and useful consultations from national experts on pressure sores.

I believe we should listen to these stories. Somewhere along the route of reform too many of us have lost sight of the simpler principles and sensible practices that provide the foundations for rapid improvement. Somewhere along the route we have become tangled in approaches and initiatives that do not make deep sense to us because they do not make sense at all. We have the capability to make incredible improvements in the care we give, but my father and thousands like him will continue to lie beyond the reach of that capacity unless we shift gears and head back toward sense.

Here are five changes we need:

1. *We must change our focus from integrating structures to integrating experiences.*

I have serious doubts as to whether the current wave of mergers, acquisitions, and reorganizations now sweeping almost every large market in health care will matter at all to persons like my father unless the leaders so engaged build on their new structures by asking themselves a simple question: Why should the people of this community—those who are sick or those who may become sick—care that this change in structure or ownership has occurred? The answer, if it is honest, must relate to improving the experiences of care. As structures, our new "integrated delivery systems" should not be end points in themselves. They matter in the long run only as foundations for redesigning the processes of care so that patients get better help. In my father's transition among facilities—from hospital to nursing home to rehabilitation facility to his home—he was in the care of five different teams of physical therapists. Five different evaluation forms were completed, with five different recommendations, for five separate fees. The only evident transfer of evaluation documents occurred when I drove to the hospital, picked up a copy of the evaluation, and took it to the nursing home. There I was told, "We never use outside evaluations."

By contrast, integrating appointment processes in one portion of one region of Kaiser Permanente has reduced the waiting list for healthy-adult appointments from two thousand to zero in three months, while the total clinical staff required to supply those appointments decreased by 4 percent.

2. *We must learn to use measurement for improvement, not for judgment.*

The dominant use of measurement in health care systems is what I call "measurement for judgment," not "measurement for improvement." Report cards, benchmark comparisons, accreditation processes, and employer-based performance surveys are all inspection-based systems seeking data that can be used to make choices. The underlying strategy is to improve through culling, and it is a distant second-best to the real improvement that comes only through continuous effort and pervasive change. I fear the rush to collect information whose main effect will be to quell aspiration and invite dishonesty. Learning begins with curiosity, and curiosity is never totally safe. Public reports on health care performance may help to motivate change, but the responsibility to make changes that will actually help patients cannot be placed outside the system; it is those of us who are inside who must change.

Contrast reliance on culling with the approach that Bill Nugent describes as a support system for his team's dramatic improvements in cardiac outcomes over the past two years. In a recent letter to me Nugent wrote, "By continuously tracking our outcomes, we have found it much easier to organize ourselves. . . . We needed earlier warnings of statistically real problems. . . . We now rely on control charts . . . used to track input variables ([such as] patient demographics), process variables ([such as] intubation and length of stay), and outcome variables ([such as] mortality, morbidity, patient satisfaction, functional health). All this is now reported back in the form of a cardiac surgical instrument panel. In sum, I have worked to develop effective ways to collect high-quality clinical data and, more importantly, to use that data to improve outcomes."

3. *We must move beyond a naive search for best practices to a much healthier mode of learning from one another.*

I recently asked my fifteen-year-old daughter, Jessica, an avid horseback rider, whether it would help her to see a video of the

Olympic gold medalist in dressage so she could copy her. "I'd enjoy it," said Jessica, "but it wouldn't help me much." Why? "Because what I need to learn right now isn't what she would show me."

This sensibility—seeing learning as a process, not a goal—characterizes the persons involved in the best improvements in health care. In reducing the rate of pressure sores by 80 percent at LDS Hospital, Carol Ashton did not begin by seeking the lowest rates in the nation and then simply copying the practices used to achieve these. Instead, she began by seeking knowledge, help, and insights and by involving her own colleagues in that undertaking. Hers was a step-by-step process, with infinite respect for the imagination and wisdom of the other adults with whom she worked. Members of Ashton's team avidly looked for ideas from outside their own system, but the solutions were inevitably and powerfully their own. And because the solutions were their own, they worked.

4. *We must shift our thinking from reduction of local cost to reduction of total cost.*

At Bethany Hospital, the dramatic improvements in outcomes for adults with asthma were accomplished in a resource-starved institution that treats the poorest of populations. Ask Carolyn Jackson how it was done and she will begin by describing new initiatives in patient education, testing, and information systems. It will be impossible to understand how this inner-city hospital could possibly find the resources to improve until you hear Jackson make the case, as she did to her own managers and clinicians, on hard facts about total costs and benefits. "We pay now," she says, "or we definitely pay later." This was the argument, supported by data inside the hospital, that her team developed; but putting it into practice required a leadership that listened and was able to think about now and later at the same time.

I am troubled by the focus on reducing lengths of hospital stay as an end in itself. Deming warned against numerical goals, and this is one. We need to keep our minds on total costs, and it may even be that an extra day in the hospital is the best investment. We will miss that possibility if we fail to look for it. Integrated delivery systems may have a better chance of unifying views of cost, but that unifying will require many departures from classic, fragmenting assumptions about how budgets are made and monitored.

5. *We must compete against disease, not against one another.*

We have very little to rely on nowadays other than one another. I called a hospital in Houston, Texas, last year to learn about its allegedly successful innovations in pneumonia care and was told that the gains were enormous but that the methods could not be reported in public—excellent pneumonia care offered the hospital local competitive advantage. No wonder people feel confused! The enemy is disease. The competition that matters is against disease, not one another (a phrase I borrow from Dr. Paul Batalden of Dartmouth Medical School). The purpose is healing.

On my drive to work I see billboard after billboard with silly rhymes urging me to join one health maintenance organization or another; many of these organizations are distinguishable only by their logos, and they often use the very same physicians and hospitals. Every dollar of this meaningless, competitive showmanship is waste. Every beautifully printed sales brochure is care denied someone. The greatest confusion in this terribly confused year of market reform is that we think we will succeed by overcoming one another. My father does not care. He is in bed with a pressure sore, staring at a wheelchair he does not need, and living with the undeserved memory of insult, delay, and medically induced coma.

Here, again, in summary, is my agenda:

Integrate the experiences of those for whom we care.

Measure widely so we can learn to get better.

Teach one another.

Reduce the costs of the whole, not its parts.

Compete against disease and cooperate in doing so.

I propose again that we take aim where it matters. Would you consider me too self-centered if I called upon you to take steps— tomorrow morning—in honor of my father, having heard his story—the result of which will be that the story need be told no more? Pressure sores are the enemy. Stop them. Errors in drug use are the enemy. Stop them. Fragmentation is the enemy. It creates waste, cost, and disrespect. Stop it.

If we cannot work together on improvements that matter to the people who call upon us for help, then I reject your restructuring, I dismiss your mergers, I doubt your integrated system, I deplore your report card. These are only games. It was my father this time, but next time it will be your father, and then you, and then your child. I have heard it said by cynics that the quality of medical care would be far better and the hazards far less if physicians, like pilots, were passengers in their own airplanes. We are.

May I ask you to join me in a toast to my father? A pledge. An IOU on some promises due him. Not just for his sake, but for our own.

Dad, you will never walk again, but I pledge to you that I will help others to walk. I cannot take away the pain from your legs, but I promise to keep others out of pain. I cannot give you back the dignity you lost by waiting unanswered in the corridors and rooms where you should have found help, but I promise you that others will not wait and that they will be answered. I cannot undo your days of confusion from too much medication, or your weeks of frustrating spasm from too little, but I promise that others will get the treatments they need—no more and no less. I cannot explain why your savings from forty years of hard work are melting in one-tenth the time into a cauldron of undecipherable bills—why your wheelchair costs $6,000 and your hip repair costs more dollars than the house you raised us in; why you have insurance for your fruitless electromyogram, but not for the kind lady at home who softens the pain in your pressure sore from midnight to dawn. I cannot explain why in three more years you will be destitute. I cannot explain the waste you now must pay for, but I promise that the hard-earned savings of others will be treated with more respect and caution. I promise you to try to make destitution neither the cause nor the consequence of disease.

To help in this, I call to your bedside people who promise too. I call Carol Ashton and Michael Morris. I call Carolyn Jackson and Bill Nugent and Terry Clemmer and Charles Guise and John Burke. I call doctors and nurses and administrators and technicians who will not agree, any more than I will agree, that what has happened to you is the best we can do or the best we should do. I call thousands whom I cannot name who know that we can be better and who intend to make it so.

Further Reading

Berwick, D. M. "Eleven Worthy Aims for Clinical Leadership of Health System Reform." *JAMA*, 1994, *272*(10), 797–802.

Deming, W. E. *Out of the Crisis*. Cambridge: Massachusetts Institute of Technology, Center for Advanced Engineering Study, 1986.

Horn, S. D., Ashton, C., and Tracey, D. M. "Prevention and Treatment of Pressure Ulcers by Protocol." In S. D. Horn and D. S. Hopkins, *Clinical Practice Improvement: A New Technology for Developing Cost-Effective Quality Health Care*. New York: Faulkner & Gray, 1994, 253–262.

Pestotnik, S. L., Classen, D. C., Evans, R. S., and Burke, J. P. "Improving Antibiotic Use: Seven-Year Results of a Process-Oriented Decision-Support System." Abstract. Proceedings of the Thirty-Third Interscience Conference on Antimicrobial Agents and Chemotherapy, New Orleans, October 17–20, 1993.

Pestotnik, S. L., Classen, D. C., Evans, R. S., and Burke, J. P. "Implementing Antibiotic Practice Guidelines Through Computer-Assisted Decision Support: Clinical and Financial Outcomes." *Annals of Internal Medicine*, 1996, *124*, 884–890.

Sandmire, H. F., and DeMott, R. K. "The Green Bay Cesarean Section Study. Part III: Falling Cesarean Birth Rates Without a Formal Curtailment Program." *American Journal of Obstetrics and Gynecology*, 1994, *170*, 1790–1802.

4

Run to Space

Commentary

Paul Batalden

Berwick's six principles for the new design of health care go right to the heart of improving health care. People in many places have used them and benefited. I wonder why we haven't been able to apply them everywhere and benefit everyone? Robert Kegan and Lisa Lahey offer a model that might help in their book, *How the Way We Talk Can Change the Way We Work: Seven Languages for Transformation.* They suggest that our best intentions don't become reality because we are engaged in a variety of daily activities that regularly get in the way of our commitments to improve. What underlie these activities are our "competing commitments." We give these commitments "trumping power" through the "big assumptions" that underpin them. These assumptions often go unexamined and untested. To try out this model, you might wish to create a matrix like the one in Table 4.1.

Do it with a good friend—someone with whom you can be completely honest, particularly about columns three (Competing Commitments) and four (Big Assumptions). If you find that common activities, commitments, or habits are at work across the six principles, you have identified areas for change that are likely to offer significant leverage in your personal change efforts. If you

Table 4.1. Identifying Areas for Personal Change Using Berwick's Six Principles.

A Better Way	Daily Actions	Competing Commitments	Big Assumptions
1. Reduce waste in all of its forms.			
2. Study and apply the principle of continuous flow.			
3. Reduce demand.			
4. Plot measurements related to aims over time.			
5. Match capacity to demand.			
6. Cooperate.			

learn that what is true for you is also true for your friend or trusted colleague, you can work on common or concurrent efforts and thus encourage each other. If you both work in the same context and find common obstacles, or assumptions that are not supportable, you are likely to learn about how the organizational culture in which you work either contributes to or handicaps your efforts to change and improve.

The heart of this insight seems to be related to making *implicit* inferential processes *explicit*. By doing so, it becomes easier to examine these processes, to test their validity, and to have meaningful conversation about them.

Knowing what prevents us from changing is not the same as doing something about it, but if we can identify the competing commitments and the underlying assumptions, we can attempt to validate them and test changes in them. It often works best to start with testing a small change in a big assumption. By empirically demonstrating to ourselves that our competing commitments and their assumptions don't deserve their favored status, we can find new possibilities for taking action on the sound principles that Berwick suggests.

Further Reading

Kegan, R., and Lahey, L. *How the Way We Talk Can Change the Way We Work: Seven Languages for Transformation*. San Francisco: Jossey-Bass, 2000.

Run to Space

7th Annual National Forum on Quality Improvement in Health Care

Orlando, Florida, December 3, 1995

These are the Angels (Figure 4.1). I am their coach. Because I am hopelessly confused about where we are currently headed in health care, I thought I might spend my hour with you avoiding the topic. I prefer, with your permission, to focus on fourth grade girls' soccer instead of on health care improvement. Those of you who want a refund can form a line outside the door.

Here are some basic principles of fourth grade girls' soccer:

1. It is primarily an educational and developmental undertaking in which self-esteem, basic skill building, and fun are regarded as extremely important—just behind winning at all costs.

2. Coaches are in charge of snacks.

3. Parents of different teams have to stand on opposite sides of the field at games, for the good of all concerned.

4. All teams must be named after benign supernatural creatures—angels, spirits, pixies, and so forth—or after small rodents—gerbils, squirrels, and chipmunks, but not rats.

This is my preparation to be a coach. My motivation is to try to put behind me my entire childhood of athletic incompetence, in which my most vivid memory is of Jimmy Golub walking up to me silently in the eighth inning of a Little League Baseball game in

Keynote speech presented at the 7th Annual National Forum on Quality Improvement in Health Care, Orlando, Florida, December 3, 1995.

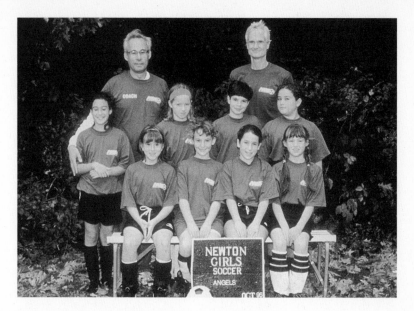

Figure 4.1. The Angels.

which my record of strikeouts as a batter remained unblemished and asking me softly and with genuine curiosity, "Why do you do this?"

At any rate, I have been determined this season to lead the Angels well. Here is my strategy.

I began with laissez-faire. Empowerment. Great kids, enthusiastic, early purchasers of shin guards. My job was to let them loose to do what they came to do. I empowered them. My speech at the beginning of our first game (against the Pixies) was simple: "You're professionals. You know what to do. Go for it." Results: Angels 1, Pixies 4.

I elected to switch my strategy. Perhaps, I thought, these girls—women—are not as motivated as I had initially believed. We need a results orientation. I began pointing to the scoreboard repeatedly in game two. I gave them feedback. When they scored a goal, I yelled from the sidelines, "You scored a goal! You scored a goal!" When they missed, I yelled, "You missed! Next time, don't miss!" They looked at me. We lost: Angels 1, Gremlins 2.

No more Mr. Nice Guy. I had parents on my back. People were making unkind analogies to the Red Sox. Girls began bringing homework to practice. We were in crisis. It was time for performance pay, except that, of course, paying fourth graders was illegal. So I used Hershey Bars. I put the halftime cookies at stake. No score: no cookies. Score: Hershey Bar. Simple, direct, informative. We lost: Angels 2, Marmots 3.

The team rewards were of course insufficient motivation. Report cards became individualized. At each quarter I posted the scores by individual players, protecting their anonymity, of course, by calling Lauren "Player A," Meg "Player B," and so forth. Each player got individualized feedback, with her row highlighted in yellow marker pen. Results were immediate but unanticipated. Lauren vomited. Julia's mother called to tell me that Julia had had a sore throat and I should adjust her score. Everyone tried to score, and no one passed, until I gave half-credit for assists, in which case everyone passed (since assists were easier) and no one tried to score. No one would play goalie, and when I said I really did value goalies, they said, "Yeah, right," pointing to the scoring sheet. They insisted that I case-mix adjust the individual scores according to the competence of the other team, the weather, and so forth. I said, "You don't get the point; we have to beat them no matter who they are." I decided to try to move to a different strategy when Lizzie's father, a construction contractor, showed up at game five with a bulldozer, saying he was going to level the playing field. Angels 0, Gerbils 6.

Guidelines were the answer. I realized—how could I have been so stupid?—that the real problem was lack of standards for plays. We soon produced our first soccer guideline (Figure 4.2.A). We soon revised it (Figure 4.2.B). Then, based on our scouting of the Gerbil benchmark, we realized we needed some branching logic (Figure 4.2.C). We then lost again.

In game eight I began to learn something. It started when Rebecca came up to me at halftime and said, "I'm sick of losing."

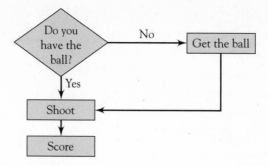

Figure 4.2.A. Soccer Guideline.

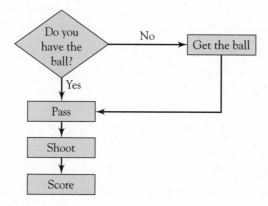

Figure 4.2.B. Revised Soccer Guideline.

"Oh, yeah?" I said, sipping my cappuccino. "If you're so sick of losing, why not win?"

"I'd like to," she said, "but we need coaching."

"What do you mean?" I asked. "I have been coaching you for two months."

"Well," said Lizzie, "not exactly. I mean, do you know how to play soccer?"

"You're the player," I said, a little sweaty under my collar. "I'm just the coach."

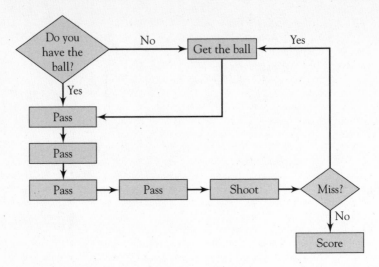

Figure 4.2.C. Soccer Guideline with Branching Logic: The Gerbil Benchmark.

"Well," said Lizzie, "*why* are you the coach? You mean, you're the coach and you don't know how to play the game?"

"Sure I do," I said. "I point out the scoreboard, I motivate, I make guidelines, I tell you pass-pass-pass-shoot. That's my job."

"You don't get it," said Lizzie. "It doesn't help me when you yell, 'pass-pass-pass-shoot.' You have to tell me *how*. How do you play soccer?"

It got me thinking. How do you play soccer?

I have had the honor of delivering a series of speeches at our National Forums through the years. Some of you may recall those speeches. Some of you may even have studied them. To you I say, "Get a life." In those speeches I have sometimes talked about the why of what we do. I have talked about my patients, about the unmet social need for our help, and last year, about my own father—a victim of deficient care. In other Forum speeches I have talked about what we could make better. Two years ago I set out for your consideration eleven aims—eleven areas in which our current performance bears little relationship to what we know, scientifically, is possible to achieve.

The Institute for Healthcare Improvement has in the past year organized a set of Collaboratives—we call it the Breakthrough Series—in which organizations that have the will and the spirit to set in place improvement agendas for these and other aims get a chance to help one another and to draw upon the experience and advice of the best experts in the nation. Three Collaboratives are now under way—on reducing cesarean section rates, on improving asthma care, and on reducing waits and delays throughout the care system—and several more will begin soon—on reducing medication errors and other hazards in medical settings, on reducing costs and improving outcomes in adult intensive care units, on reducing costs and improving outcomes in cardiovascular surgery, and on improving care for low back pain.

Working with these Collaboratives has already taught me a lot that I did not know about improvement, and I hope all of you will eventually join one or another of them to learn more yourself. But the biggest lesson of all has been the same one I learned from my fourth-grade team: to improve soccer, you have to know how to play soccer. To improve care, you have to know how to deliver care. And to an extent greater than I realized until recently, the job of envisioning the new system—the job of knowing and explaining better ways to do work—is nondelegable. That is, just as clarifying organizational aim is the duty and privilege of leaders, so is clarifying and insisting upon major principles of design for the system of work. Leaders must be prepared to assert not only *what* must be accomplished, but also *how* it can be accomplished. I do not think this is a comfortable message for senior leaders to hear. Many would rather rely on simpler notions of "empowerment," in which the workers—clinicians and others—are expected to invent new ways to work. This, in my opinion, is not an effective route to the redesigns that our aims require. Leaders have to be able to *coach* on methods.

We have talked about *why* we should improve, and we have talked about *what* we can improve. This is the year of *how*. Let me explain.

As many of you know, the American automobile industry has experienced a major turnaround in the current decade. Fifteen years ago, the big three auto companies in this nation were, in their own ways, each on death's doorstep. In 1980, Ford was losing billions of dollars each year, Chrysler was approaching bankruptcy, and General Motors had calculated less than a five-year future before it was out of business. Last year, all three companies made unprecedented profits, and there is objective evidence that American vehicles are fully the equal of Japanese in quality and, protectionism aside, lower in cost. How did they get there?

The answer is not simple, but it has a simple form. To a large extent, the ongoing rescue of the American automobile industry, though by no means complete, occurred because that industry figured out a better way to make a car.

Let me repeat: they figured out a better way to make a car.

Let me spell out what this means. This means that if in, say, 1975 you had visited a Ford plant and studied the basic processes of production, you would have found a series of activities informed by an underlying series of premises about the right way to make a car. If you had asked about inventory levels, they would have said, "We keep our inventories high so as to protect the production line against shortages." If you had asked about inspection of incoming parts, they would have said, "We carefully inspect everything we receive from suppliers so as to ensure quality at the receiving dock." If you had asked about turnover of machines from one product to another—such as converting a sheet metal stamping machine from economy model doors to luxury model doors—they would have said, "Conversion takes days. Therefore, we book long runs. No use stopping the line for repeated switchovers from vehicle to vehicle." If you had asked about suppliers, they would have said, "We keep them at bay. Competitive bidding—that's the way to keep them on their toes." With each answer they would have shown their conviction about the right way to make a car.

If, however, you visited the same plant today and asked the same questions, here are the answers you would get. Inventories: "Not high, low. We aim for zero inventories, if possible. We aim for delivery of what we need just in time—that's best for both cost and quality." If you asked about inspection at the receiving dock they would say, "We are trying to eliminate it. We qualify our suppliers so that we don't need to inspect. Inspection isn't a reflection of quality; it's a surrender to poor quality." Machine turnover? Fundamentally new. "We used to take two days to change over," they would say. "Now we take two hours. As a result, we can manage very short runs instead of long runs. In fact," they would tell you, "we are soon approaching the car made to order. Production runs of size one. That's where we are headed." What about suppliers? "Fewer and fewer," they would say. "Simple competitive bidding is long gone. We want good prices, of course, but we make more money on relationships. We want partners for the long haul."

Now, a couple of points about this second visit are worth noting. First, in many cases not only would the current rule have been regarded as undesirable at visit one, but it would also have been considered impossible. Short production runs? Poppycock. Give up bidding? Silly. Two-hour turnover? In your dreams! Inspection is the lifeblood of quality. That's what you would have heard.

In the twenty-year interval, you see, not only the practice changed—the theory changed. The convictions about the correct way to organize work changed. The very definition of idealized production changed.

Contrast this with my pediatric office. I see patients in a very good HMO, but I would like you to imagine that you videotaped a day in my practice as a doctor in 1979, when I first started, and then taped me again last week as I saw patients. If you ran both tapes blind, could you tell the difference? Many of you in the audience know the answer. The answer is, "No." By and large, I make care now just like I made care twenty years ago.

But the answer is not always no. Take the boy with asthma who I walked in upon as the triage doctor several weeks ago. He was the four-year-old son of an inner-city teenage mother. I had not met either of them ever before. He was breathing with great difficulty, and twenty, ten, or five years ago I would have simply picked up the phone and called the ambulance to take him to the hospital emergency room for admission. But here is what happened instead.

When I walked into the room, his mother handed me her written record of his home nebulizer treatments of the prior twenty-four hours, administered by her. She told me what his peak expiratory flow rate (which she measured at home) was before and after each treatment, and she gave me a complete history of each of his medications. She recommended the next medication to try and suggested that I call her asthma outreach nurse on the nurse's cellular phone. At about the same time, the allergy chief knocked on the door of my office, having popped down from his office one floor above; he already knew that the child was coming in because the asthma outreach nurse had phoned him. He handed me a vial of the new medication that was usually effective in this child and on the spot arranged for a follow-up phone call later that afternoon. Two hours later the child was not in an emergency room on his way to a hospital bed; instead he was at home, breathing fine, and watching Barney on TV.

None of this could have been easily imagined ten years ago— neither home nebulization, nor the mother's skill in measurement of flow rate, nor the availability of an outreach nurse on a cellular phone, nor an allergy chief one floor up who regarded popping in as part of his job, nor the record system that kept us all on the same page. This is a change in rules of play every bit as fundamental as the better way to make a car. It is a new system, founded on new principles of how work is done.

A new system. A change. The production method was unprecedented, and therefore we could achieve an unprecedented result.

In the world of automobiles, some call the new methods "lean production." General Motors has given me permission to show you this chart (Figure 4.3), which diagrams in more detail than you might wish some of the core elements of lean production. These principles are now the assumptions, and did not used to be, of the best makers of cars in the world. These principles are better than the old ones, and if you do not use them or beat them today, you die. Here are the principles I spoke about earlier, described in the terms that General Motors uses: low inventories achieved with "pull systems" of just-in-time delivery, small production runs achieved through quick set-up times, supplier development as a major agenda. This is now the proper way, not the old way, to make a car.

It works in soccer, too. One example of a good production principle in fourth grade soccer is this: "Run to space." Fourth grade girls tend to come in clumps. If they are not in a clump, they will try to get into a clump. On a soccer field, this means that one can usually find five of any six Angels all trying to kick the ball from the same place at the same time. Gerbils will also be there. Girls in such circumstances get kicked more often than the ball does.

Unclumping is a good idea. The way to say it to a ten-year-old is, "Run to space." That means, whether you think it is rational at the time or not, try not to run to where the ball is. Run to where it isn't. Run to where nobody is. If you do that, a surprisingly large number of times, the ball will pop out to you, all alone, and you will get a chance to pass or shoot. A chance you won't have in a clump of rodents.

To make it clearer to my team, I said, "Angels are poison. If you are anywhere near another Angel, they will kill you. If you don't want to die, run to space." They loved it, and spread out immediately all over the field. One even went over to the next field. What a coach!

Now, in health care we are not unfamiliar with the idea of new principles of work. In the decades of the 1970s, we did adopt one, which was to move our care from inpatient to outpatient settings. Tell a doctor in 1965 that a hernia repair or tonsillectomy or even

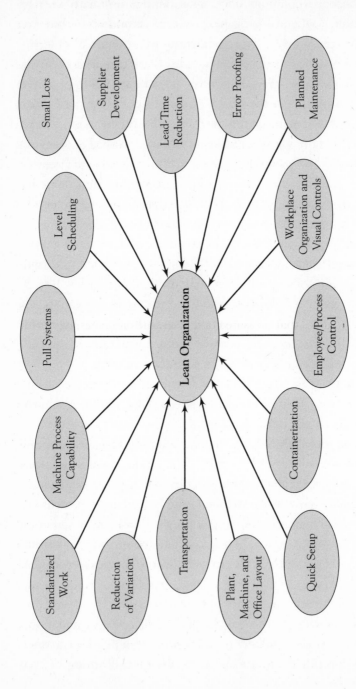

Figure 4.3. Lean Production.
Source: General Motors.

an endoscopy would be done in an outpatient unit with a patient who would go home after six or twelve hours and you would have been certified as crazy. Today, to do otherwise is crazy.

More recently we have exploded in health care with two other principles—and we have bet a bundle on them. These principles are guidelines and feedback on performance data. For some reason or other, we have grasped the idea that we ought to write down specifications for our work, and that we ought to issue performance data in various versions, in an effort to improve what we do.

I am not sure exactly where these ideas came from. Nor do I oppose them. We have some evidence that both have effects and that, in the black box of health care work, both lead doctors and others to change what they do in useful ways. A recent review in *The Lancet* shows encouragingly that in fifty-five of fifty-nine published studies of the effects of guidelines, the care process did change significantly in the direction of the guideline, and in nine of eleven studies that measured outcomes, the outcomes improved.[1] The review also showed some ways to make guidelines especially effective: develop them locally, train in specific ways, and invoke them at the time and place of care, perhaps with automated reminder systems. There is similar encouraging information about how feedback can help.

But on the whole I think that guidelines and feedback are only poor second cousins to a fully developed notion of new ways to provide health care. They lack the theoretical power we would need to really remake our work. To achieve leverage in change, we need better leveraged concepts—ideas and principles for the design of the work of care that are as powerful in health care as the principles of lean production have been proving to be in manufacturing. In fact, I would suggest that we need some of the same principles as in lean production.

Let me spell out some examples—six ideas, in particular, that represent for me appropriate foundations of design for the era of change that will be responsive to the new context of care.

1. *Reduce waste in all of its forms.*

I believe that we have not yet scratched the surface of the opportunity for waste reduction in health care. In the aggressive search for cost reductions, I have seen only a few health care organizations take seriously the notion of waste in a broad way, building their business strategies on this foundation. By contrast, leading companies have built a large portion of their strategies for improvement around deep notions of the nature of waste and the importance of its continual reduction. Here is a list of types of waste (Figure 4.4) used by General Motors (GM) in its fast-track improvement process (called PICOS, a Spanish term for "peak of the mountains"). This list shows how broad the concept of waste can be. Professor Harry Roberts at the University of Chicago, more than a casual student of health care, has suggested that as much as 95 percent of job effort in some categories constitutes waste.[2]

Let me not leave this idea vague in health care terms. I am fond of one particular example of waste that was revealed by a study at the Kapiolani Medical Center in Honolulu, Hawaii, in late 1994. They studied gowning in newborn intensive care units (NICUs), which was costing the hospital $120,000 per year. Gowns are supposed to protect newborns from infections imported from the out-

- Inventory (documents, equipment, supplies)
- Overproduction
- Complexity
- Handoffs
- Correction (inspection, rework)
- Movement of materials and information
- Unnecessary processing
- Waiting
- Motion of people

Figure 4.4. Types of Waste.
  Source: General Motors.

side world. The problem is, there is precious little evidence that gowns work. The investigators tried an eight-month experiment: two months of gowning followed by two months without gowning and so on, and they cultured their NICU babies extensively, looking for pathogens as well as for infections and deaths. The result, as in twelve of the fourteen prior published studies of gowning, was negative. Gowning does not protect babies. The $120,000 and the associated time and complexity were waste.[3]

I have often wondered since about the following experiment. Suppose I had counted the number of NICUs in the United States and Canada using gowns in, say, July 1994, three months before the Kapiolani study, and then suppose I had counted again in January 1995, three months after the study. Would the numbers differ? Most of those who know health care up close would predict that the answer would be no. We do not choose to change, even when the evidence of waste is there. We lack, I think, a sense of waste. We do not hunt it out. We accept it. As Dr. Joseph Juran puts it, we "disconnect the alarm." As a result, for every thousand hospitals that continue to gown, we waste $120,000 times 1,000, or $120,000,000 every year.

Suppose we became students and hunters of waste in its relatively pure forms. What would we find? Dr. Johan Thor and I identified more than fifty specific wasteful activities over the past several weeks, based upon a rapid review of recently published literature from mainstream, peer-reviewed journals and of the reports of colleagues at the Mayo Clinic and Virginia Mason Medical Center. These activities could be stopped tomorrow in your health care organization, probably without harming anyone, except, of course, for the pain involved in reallocation of energies or reductions in force that are unhappily implied by some. The ideas include both simple waste, in which something like gowning could be stopped (Figure 4.5.A), and substitutions, in which a less expensive drug, test, or procedure could be substituted without harm for a more expensive one (Figure 4.5.B). The ideas are ready for you to test

- Gowning in NICUs
- Yearly sports examination in junior high school
- Routine type and Coombs' on cord blood
- Routine changes of ventilator circuits
- Unjustified blood transfusions
- MMR "desensitization" in egg allergy
- Routine screening urinalysis in children
- Patient-specific inpatient menus

Figure 4.5.A. Examples of Waste.

- Asthma outreach programs
- Short-course UTI therapy
- Risk scores before ankle and knee X-rays
- Miconazole for dermatophyte infections
- Simple antibiotics for otitis media
- Postop fever algorithm in total hip patients

Figure 4.5.B. Examples of Smart Substitution.

locally if you care about reducing waste. How many of you will cease gowning before the next National Forum?

The choice is not about whether or not to reduce our costs, or about whether or not to downsize. It is about how to do so in the ways that are least harmful to our mission and to those who are supposed to benefit from our work. It is about how to preserve and improve what is valuable, instead of discarding value along with waste in blunt, mindless budget cuts.

A conviction that waste is pervasive, an understanding of its nature and types, a commitment to find it, and a commitment to stop it quickly are all part of the new principles of lean production, and they ought to be principles—fundamental and universal principles—in systems of care.

At the Mayo Clinic, a team headed by Dr. Michael Ebersold identified tests and equipment wasted in the care of orthopedic patients. For decades blood had been typed and crossed for transfusion but was never used. They stopped it. Postoperative X-rays for joint replacement had been done routinely by an orthopedic group. They never used them. They stopped it. Routine preoperative tests were unnecessary for large classes of patients. They stopped using them. I am not saying that you should consider copying the Mayo Clinic—unless, of course, you respect them.

2. *Study and apply the principle of continuous flow.*

It took a genius—Taiichi Ohno—to develop the core theories of production that today underlie so-called just-in-time production processes, also called Kanban systems or the Toyota production process.[4] What Ohno noticed was that the absence of continuous flow was in itself a deep form of waste. The price of interrupted flow was either inventory (stacks of unused things that might sometime be used) or waits (as people needing things turned to empty bins or people needing service cooled their heels). Ohno, as I understand his thought process, began to imagine production as a kind of river—a river in which no molecule of water ever waited, no molecule ever stacked up (except at a dam), and each molecule filled the space of the one ahead exactly when it was pulled to that space as the preceding particle left it. His vision transformed the notion of production from a push system—making it and passing it along—to a pull system in which the need "pulled" the supply only when, and exactly when, the need was there.

The realization of this concept was astounding. One measure is inventory turns—the speed with which an item received from a supplier is used in the actual product.

My colleague and mentor Blan Godfrey shared with me the data shown here (Figure 4.6) on what modern manufacturers are achieving today in inventory turns. By some measures, modern use of continuous flow reduces inventory by two or more orders of magnitude.

Standard:	4 per year
Best practice:	>100 per year
Possible:	16 per day
Inventory reduction:	41%–82%

Figure 4.6. Inventory Turns.

We do not understand continuous flow and its immense potential in health care. Our hospitals and clinics are to a large extent areas for inventory and waiting—stacks of things and people idle while they await other things and people. Waiting rooms, holding areas, storage spaces, bins—stacks and delays.

It does not need to be that way. Just as it would be a revolution in our thinking to identify waste in all of its forms, so it would be a revolution to understand that waiting and stacks are symptoms of systems incapable of smooth, continuous flow. Every time we process things in a batch—forms, people, equipment, appointments—we are surrendering to waste.

I recently saw a project from Wesley Medical Center in Wichita, Kansas, where continuous flow principles are being taken very seriously indeed. A pharmacy project using small batches instead of large ones reduced total IV fluid use by 17 percent and returns for credit (a measure of defect) by 24 percent. These reductions only begin to account for the financial and other benefits, however. Continuous flow systems are cheaper for everyone, and better for customers.

A health care leader who wanted to insist that continuous flow become a characteristic of a system could take a simple beginning step by walking around looking for waits and batches and then asking how each could be removed without additional resources. Such a leader would soon be saving millions of dollars and improving care at the same time.

3. *Reduce demand.*

For decades I have heard providers of care complain bitterly about unrealistic patient demands for unnecessary care: the mother who insists on a CAT scan for her child with a headache; the anxious man who insists on cardiac imaging for vague chest pain. Yet for every hundred such complaints, I have seen barely one wholehearted effort to really change demand in safe and respectful ways. We have not developed sound ways to help our patients seek their own self-interest, and we have allowed the public to proceed on the dangerous, toxic, and expensive assumption that more is better.

The evidence is often otherwise. I have had the pleasure for the past five years of serving as vice chair of the U.S. Preventive Services Task Force, a quasi-public advisory panel for the U.S. Department of Health and Human Services equipped with brilliant and committed staff, with the sole charge of reviewing the scientific evidence in more than six thousand journal papers for and against almost two hundred clinical preventive practices.[5] This is the second incarnation of the Task Force; the first group published its conclusions about 169 clinical preventive services in 1989.[6]

The reviews and assessments are fair and careful, and I can tell you—but you can read it for yourself as well—that very few of the practices reviewed, even common ones, make it over the hurdle of sound scientific evidence. Yet many of these practices continue, without evidentiary support, in common use. Sometimes the reasons for continuation are good. But often they are not.

Leaders at Group Health Cooperative of Puget Sound took managing demand seriously when they noted the overuse of PSA (prostate-specific antigen) screening tests compared to recommendations of the U.S. Preventive Services Task Force. With a carefully crafted combination of education, feedback, and so-called academic detailing, they reduced the proportion of their own primary care providers misusing the test to 3 percent, while surveys in the greater

Seattle area showed that 80 percent of non-Group Health Cooperative primary care providers in that region continued to follow the outmoded practice.

Here is the challenge: for useless care, develop and improve methods to help the public understand the futility and, in view of the possibility of error, the complications and hazards that unneeded care can introduce. I personally regard the continuing use of ineffective care—tests, procedures, drugs, and visits—less as testimony to the insatiability of our patients and their families than as testimony to our lack of commitment to the serious redesign and continuous improvement of processes that shape their expectations and understanding of what helps and what does not help. At best we have erected barriers to entry—co-payments, deductibles, rules, precertifications, waiting lists, quotas, and queues—all of which are unpleasant to some degree, and many of which cannot distinguish between needed services and wasteful ones.

4. *Plot measurements related to aims over time.*

This simple principle seems hardly to stand by itself as an important guide to the work of health care in the future; but do not be deceived. Plotting measurement over time turns out, in my view, to be one of the most powerful devices we have for systemic learning. In fact, no less a thinker than Walter Shewhart—founding theorist of statistical process control—built his major contributions around the design and interpretation of simple plots of data over time. In its fullest form this became the control chart, which today is still the bedrock technique for process control.[7]

Several important things happen when you plot data over time. First, you have to ask what data to plot. In the exploration of the answer you begin to clarify aims, and also to see the system from a wider viewpoint. Where are the data? What do they mean? To whom? Who should see them? Why? These are questions that integrate and clarify aims and systems all at once. Second, you get a leg up on improvement. When important indicators are continuously monitored, it becomes easier and easier to study the effects of innovation in real time, without deadening delays for setting up measurement systems or obsessive collections during baseline periods of inaction. Tests of change get simpler to interpret when we use time as a teacher. The plot over time is a powerful supplement to the randomized trial.

Tom Nighswander and his colleagues in Anchorage, Alaska, have been tackling a tough problem—death rates in the first year of life in high-risk Native American populations—through an innovative outreach program they call *Nutaqsiivik*, which is an Eskimo word for "renewal." To track the effect of the program, they follow, among other things, a simple measure of "time between postneonatal deaths." Because they track this time, they can study the effects of their own program much more easily than if they had to set up a new data system or a randomized trial every time they made a change.

So convinced am I of the power of this principle of tracking over time that I would suggest this: If you follow only one piece of advice from this lecture when you get home, pick a measurement you care about and begin to plot it regularly over time. You won't be sorry.

5. *Match capacity to demand.*

I already touched on this idea when I discussed continuous flow earlier, because these are related principles. But I want to emphasize this one even more. Much of the waste and delay in health care comes from mismatches between supply and demand; in particular, we tend to maintain high capacities in order to meet sporadic demands. We used to say in training that we doctors were sitting in emergency rooms waiting for the busload of hemophiliacs to hit the tree. It sounds safe and prudent to prepare for the onslaught. We are there when you need us.

Gradually, however, such "buffered" systems become inefficient. Idle time becomes an entitlement. We recall the intermittent surge of demand instead of the long intervals of waiting. We remember the time we ran out of something, then increase our stocks even more to prevent that from ever happening again. We imagine what could happen, and we staff to relieve our fear.

No truly modern system of work does that anymore. Buffers cost too much and are the protection of last resort. What works better is to use information to make predictions. With predictions we can allocate resources more intelligently prospectively. The tricks are two.

First, we need to be able to predict by having data about demand and supply, and to allocate what we have easily and quickly in response.

Second, and much harder to learn, we need to give up the idea that the core system must have the capacity to meet the special need. The core system must have the capacity to meet the core need; for the special need, we should aim for special systems. That is why we have disaster manuals in hospitals, instead of always staffing for a disaster that might happen someday. That is why airports are under special security rules when a terrorist is on the loose, instead of having the most stringent rules in effect all the time.

The new principle of production is this: Measure cycle time, measure demand, measure supply, make a prediction, and allocate to meet the core need 70 percent or 80 percent of the time. Develop special, intermittent systems to meet the special, intermittent needs.

In one of our Breakthrough Series projects we are focusing on reducing delays and we are using principles of continuous flow to advantage. One related principle is simple: Predict demand and allocate supply to anticipate it. That idea alone led to the success experienced in a urology clinic (Figure 4.7), which reduced its waiting time for appointments by 80 percent without adding any staff, space, or equipment. The staff did just four basic things: they measured supply, measured demand, made a small predictive model, and allocated clinician time according to the model.

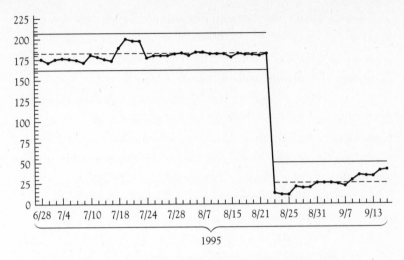

Figure 4.7. Waiting Time for Appointments in Urology Clinic.

6. Cooperate.

Let me propose the principle of cooperation as a new foundation for our work. New, you say? What is new about cooperation?

I suggest that cooperation at the level at which we need to learn and practice it would be new in health care, and furthermore, among all of the principles of lean production that we could adopt in our system, this principle—cooperate—is the prince of principles, in some sense the ruler and enabler of all the other principles that matter.

What would you say if my soccer team did not cooperate? No passes, no scores. It's obvious. Cooperation and success are related.

Now, just for laughs, suppose that the soccer field suddenly burst into flames in the middle of a game between the Angels and the Marmots. Sparks and cinders everywhere. Screaming fourth-grade girls running around, brushing flames from their soccer shirts. Suddenly, a Marmot falls to the ground, ankle sprained, yelling for assistance. Katie, an Angel, rushes past her, heedless of her cries.

"Katie," I yell, "see that girl? She's injured! Help her get up and lead her off the field."

"No," says Katie, "not on your life. She's a Marmot. I'm an Angel."

"Katie," I'd scream back, "have you lost your mind? There's a fire now. The game's off. Angels and Marmots don't matter. You're just a girl now, and so is she. New game, Katie. New rules."

Cooperation is a matter of context. Whether we see it and expect it depends on how we draw the system of relevance. A well-run cardiac resuscitation is a ballet of cooperation, role fitted perfectly to role. Prior jealousy and professional prerogatives don't matter anymore. Getting the job done matters in a system of the whole.

In health care today we are like Angels killing Marmots. Same girls, different uniforms. I have been in several American cities of similar description with the following facts in place. Several in this room will think I am speaking specifically of them, which will only make my point better.

The university hospital is in trouble. It is being cut out of the action and is a takeover target for outsiders. Training programs and research are threatened. Managed care is consolidating into a few big players, but the poor population in town is suffering a gradual withdrawal of core services. The city remains overbuilt in inpatient services, especially in high technology, with too many angiography suites, three organ transplant units when one would do, two cardiac surgery units when one would do, extra obstetrical beds and more being built. Improvement activities are somewhat secret, and one hospital will not tell another about its new methods of cost reduction in operating room care, while the second won't tell the first about how it has achieved more appropriate antibiotic use. Everyone is developing critical paths for diabetes, with mostly the same results, but redundant development continues. With managed care, capitation, and a for-profit threat looming, the field is bursting into flames.

In the privacy of their homes, each CEO says the same thing: "This is silly. We could do a lot better if we worked together, but

it's impossible." Each will quote his or her (mostly his) list of barriers to cooperation: the Federal Trade Commission (FTC), the Justice Department, a history of bad blood, "I just cannot work with
him," "I trusted him once, but never again." Each will explain why
the right thing is impossible. The soccer game goes on with the
field ablaze.

It is stupid. It is stupid activity led by very smart people. I admit
to not understanding this paradox as much as I would like to, but
underneath it all I feel a deep sense of loss and a pervasive impres-
sion that the root cause lies not in the FTC or in the payer or in the
wisdom of market logic or in the evidence of evildoing. It is rather
a matter of some missing skill, some capacity that our leaders,
despite their genius, and despite their shared good intentions overall, do not have. Once, when I asked a wise man for advice about
solving a very difficult problem that I was having with a powerful
figure in my life, he said this to me: "The solution is easy and you
know what it is. But first," he said, "you will have to jump over your
own shadow."

Jump over my own shadow. What did that mean? It meant that
the problem of cooperation was not outside of me, it was inside me.
It was a darkness made of my own ignorance and assumption, of my
own interpretations, and to be frank, of my own cowardice. To be
brave enough to reconsider. To be brave enough to trust that
another was like me. To be brave enough to abandon the familiar
pattern of accusation inside my own head, and to act in violation
of that pattern. These were my obstacles. And there was no route
to cooperation other than jumping over them.

There is a drawing in Watzlawick, Weakland, and Fisch's book,
Change, that shows two people on a sailboat, each of whom is hiked
out dangerously to either side; neither can stand upright without
cooperation.[8] To achieve that requires a succession of small, trusting steps. First one must move, then the other, then the one, and
then the other. It requires signaling through action and reciprocity
of giving. There is no other option.

Children tell a riddle. Two men are in prison in adjacent cells. Each cell is full of luscious food, but each man has his arms bound rigidly at the elbows. Unable to bend his arm to feed himself, each man is slowly starving. What should they do? The answer is surprisingly hard to get from most audiences, except from children: To survive they must feed each other.

I went into my local pizza store—Bertucci's—last year and found a poster that said, "Order a pizza and we'll deliver your video." In Knapp Video, two doors down, was the converse sign, "Order a video and Bertucci's will deliver it with your pizza." Intrigued, I phoned Mr. Knapp, a perfect stranger. He graciously took my call.

"What a nice idea," I said. "How did you pull it off? Merger? Acquisition? Restructuring? Did your boards consolidate? How long were your negotiations?"

"You must be from health care," said Mr. Knapp. "It took us fifteen minutes. I spoke to Joe, the Bertucci's manager, and we decided to do it because it made sense. Merger, schmerger."

We don't seem to get it. We cannot meet the social need for health care at our current levels of cooperation—or lack of it. Maybe we need to act more like video and pizza store managers. No organization in town is good enough or big enough to solve efficiently any of the following problems in health care, and no competitive solution that I can imagine will get us there either:

Achieving an appropriate supply of high-volume, high-technology services

Controlling the AIDS epidemic

Meeting the medical needs of poor people

Improving long-term care as a system

Developing appropriate and prudent social roles and assignments for academic medical centers, with linked resources for teaching and research

Preventing accidents and injuries at the community level

Some years ago I proposed an image for a new leadership role that would be a much more fully developed model of cooperative action at the community level than any we have yet seen, or are likely to see soon. In the hope that some day some fool place will actually try it out, let me put it before you here briefly in closing. It is a model I call, "Trusteeship for the Community."

I imagine a polity in a city, a region, or a state where my friends, the video store manager and the pizza man, suddenly have responsibility for ensuring the health of the public at a price the public can afford. They become trustees of the system as a whole and they decide to cooperate to get the job done. They make the following ten changes:

1. All boards of health care organizations are assembled into a functioning systemic board, with fiduciary responsibility to rationalize the system of care as a whole.

2. That consolidated board, in full partnership with the city, develops a set of aims for improvement of the health of the city, intending to link those aims to all subsequent organizational and systemic strategies. For everyone entrusted with the leadership of elements of that system, achievement of those aims is the job.

3. Over time, and with constant refinement, the leaders of the system develop a vision for the system that must be birthed and improved to achieve those aims. The test of the value of that system is precisely its ability to achieve those aims.

4. High technology being in oversupply, the trustees of the community agree upon the appropriate level of supply to meet the community need, and downsize the elements accordingly.

5. To minimize the pain of downsizing, and to take the fullest possible advantage of attrition and personal growth, arrangements are made for transfer of staff and professionals whenever

possible among all the components of the system, when such transfer preserves jobs and growth opportunities.

6. To accelerate system improvement, a single citywide improvement resource center is created, serving as a place where all may come together to learn from one another and from experts, and to plan local improvements.

7. To emphasize the level of commitment to aims, the trustees of the community develop a set of promises about what will be achieved and by when in cost, health status, and service quality. Progress along the dimensions of these promises is regularly measured and publicly displayed. Accountability is for the performance of the community health care system as a whole, not for comparison among parts.

8. Universal access is included among the promises.

9. The trustees make a commitment to a 30 percent reduction in the total burden of illness (cost of care plus economic consequences of disease) within five years of inception of the community-wide system effort. Payers promise to put 50 percent of the economic savings into a community development fund to support better schools.

10. To build their will for cooperation, entity CEOs begin random intermittent rotations among facilities. At unpredictable times, spaced about three years apart, the CEO of facility X becomes CEO of facility Y, the CEO of facility Y becomes CEO of facility Z, and so on in a round robin.

I want us more than anything else to help each other. To do this, we need to trust, and to remember what we hold in trust.

No matter which of these principles of the new work of health care you believe, or whether you wish to identify other, better ones, my fourth-grade girls know what you need to do. To play soccer, you need to know the game; to play better, you need to know a better way to play. Our aims must be bold, and the new ways of work must be bolder still or the aims will remain out of reach. Leaders of *what* and *why* are as important as ever, but the job has matured. Leaders now must be leaders of *how*, or they will not see their teams to victory.

Run to space. The concept finally got across to my team: Angels 3, Chipmunks 1. I knew someday we would get those Chipmunks.

Notes

1. Grimshaw, J. M., and Russell, I. T. "Effect of Clinical Guidelines on Medical Practice: A Systematic Review of Rigorous Evaluations." *Lancet*, 1993, *342*(8883), 1317–1322.

2. Roberts, H. V., and Sergesketter, B. F. *Quality Is Personal: A Foundation for Total Quality Management*. New York: The Free Press, 1993, 108.

3. Pelke, S., Ching, D., Easa, D., and Melish, M. E. "Gowning Does Not Affect Colonization or Infection Rates in a Neonatal Intensive Care Unit." *Archives of Pediatrics and Adolescent Medicine*, 1994, *148*(10), 1016–1020.

4. Ohno, T. *Toyota Production System: Beyond Large-Scale Production*. Cambridge, Mass.: Productivity Press, 1988.

5. U.S. Preventive Services Task Force. *Guide to Clinical Preventive Services* (2nd ed.). Washington, D.C.: U.S. Department of Health and Human Services, 1996.

6. U.S. Preventive Services Task Force. *Guide to Clinical Preventive Services*. Washington, D.C.: U.S. Department of Health and Human Services, 1989.

7. Shewhart, W. A. *Statistical Method from the Viewpoint of Quality Control*. Washington, D.C.: Graduate School, Department of Agriculture, 1939. (Reprinted 1945.)

8. Watzlawick, P., Weakland, J. H., and Fisch, R. *Change: Principles of Problem Formation and Problem Resolution*. New York: Norton, 1988.

5

Sauerkraut, Sobriety, and the Spread of Change

Commentary

David H. Gustafson

Spreading innovations is a fundamental issue in health care. In this National Forum speech, Donald Berwick points out how desperately we need to improve health care delivery; since 1996, that need has become even more urgent, and we *know* how to improve! There exists example after example of creative innovations that have been shown to improve care dramatically. For example, we know that computer-based support systems, if appropriately designed and implemented, can improve the quality of life of breast cancer patients and enhance the recovery of patients who have had open-heart surgery. We know that improving access can reduce delays in getting appointments without increasing the workload. We know that improving patient flow in emergency rooms can reduce overcrowding and improve care.

Yet many effective improvements are never widely adopted and many disappear altogether in a short time, even in the organizations that created them. This happens even in settings where staff members want to improve, where they believe the new way is better, where management provides the resources and support needed to change. Why are we such slow learners? Are some learners faster than others, and if so, why? What characteristics of an innovation increase the likelihood that it will spread? What can be done to identify, adapt, and implement these innovations more rapidly and more permanently? What can you and I do to help spread worthwhile innovations?

In this speech Berwick tackles these issues of sustaining and spreading change in his own unique style (who would expect we could learn so much from a 250-year-old sailor, scurvy, lemons, and sauerkraut?), proposing new approaches that move beyond the literature of the field (provided so ably by gurus such as Everett Rogers, Andrew Van de Ven, and Gerald Nadler), and providing practical guidance on how to lead and support spread. He lets us see that innovations need not spread like molasses. There are things we can do now—individually, corporately, and systemically—to speed the process, and things we might do in the future to create environments where innovation can flourish.

Berwick warns us that one of the problems with a visionary is that while his or her propositions can make a lot of sense, many of them may be untested, and that testing is needed. Rogers calls this the "pro-innovation bias"—the tendency to believe that new things actually are better. Yet we all know of innovations that were implemented prematurely—for example, keeping premature infants in 100 percent oxygen, which could result in retrolental fibroplasia (an eye condition that may cause blindness). Other examples can be found in Bill Silverman's excellent book, *Where's the Evidence?*, on the premature and inappropriate introduction of innovations into medicine. So we have to be careful. Innovations need to be encouraged, but they also need to be tested carefully before full-scale implementation. This goes for Berwick's ideas as well. We need to listen carefully to his ideas, we need to encourage him to keep leading us, but we also need to test his ideas.

Improving our ability to sustain and spread change is a difficult challenge. Those who are most likely to identify innovations are treated more like lepers than leaders. To some extent, innovators bring this on themselves. They are always throwing out new ideas and wanting to try new things. Because their points of reference are more often outside the organization and even outside the industry, their loyalty is questioned. They can also be a challenge to work with. They need special care and feeding to flourish, and in today's world of limited resources and pressures to improve productivity, many managers and coworkers feel they do not have the time or energy to deal with innovators. Also, those who do try to adopt suggested innovations are often discouraged from doing so. Failing to nurture innovators can be a loss for the entire organization.

The slow spread of innovations is not a problem limited to the United States or to health care. No country or industry has solved this problem. Otherwise, Rogers' book would not be one of the most widely read books in science (now in its fifth edition), and the diffusion of innovations would not be one of the most studied fields of science. But Berwick shows us that we are up to the challenge and that there are things we as individuals can do now to make health care a role model for the rapid spread of innovations. I believe him. Read his speech, then read Rogers, Nadler, and Van de Ven. You will be richly rewarded.

Further Reading

Silverman, W. A. *Where's the Evidence? Debates in Modern Medicine*.
 New York: Oxford University Press, 1998.

Sauerkraut, Sobriety, and the Spread of Change

8th Annual National Forum on Quality Improvement in Health Care

New Orleans, Louisiana, December 4, 1996

As some of you know, I'm spending this year in Anchorage, Alaska, on a family adventure. My wife, Ann, started it. She is an innovator. She is also an environmental lawyer. For five years she headed the Environmental Protection Division of the Massachusetts Attorney General's Office. It was a wonderful job—being, as my daughter Becca says, Mother Nature's lawyer; but Ann has wanderlust, and she has always been fascinated by the Far North.

One afternoon last winter, over a margarita at a pizza restaurant, she brought up the idea: "How about taking a sabbatical next year," she said, "in Alaska?"

I panicked. I said, "There's no such thing as a sabbatical in Alaska. That is a self-contradictory expression. It's against the sabbatical code of conduct. I happen to know that the word *sabbatical* comes from the Old Norse root *sabba*, which means 'warm.' Alaska is cold."

She said, "It's a *dry* cold."

I said, "What do you mean, 'a *dry* cold'? You mean you can't have liquor with your snow? Anyway, Alaska has earthquakes. The largest earthquake in recorded history occurred in Anchorage. It was Richter 9.2."

"Nope," she said. "That was the second largest. The largest earthquake in recorded history was in Missouri, Richter 9.4." She was

Keynote speech presented at the 8th Annual National Forum on Quality Improvement in Health Care, New Orleans, Louisiana, December 4, 1996. A version of this speech was published subsequently as "Disseminating Innovations in Health Care," *JAMA*, 2003, 289(15), 1969–1975. Copyright © 2003 American Medical Association.

obviously well prepared, but I knew it was a bluff, because there was no chance at all we would move to Missouri.

"You know what I mean," I said. "Alaska had the largest *relevant* earthquake in recorded history."

Well, one thing led to another, which means Ann won, and we found ourselves in August shuttling cars between Boston and Anchorage and moving into a new house overlooking Cook Inlet. My ten-year-old daughter was quite excited. I think my seventeen-year-old daughter was excited too, but she stopped talking to us, so I don't know. The board of trustees of the Institute for Healthcare Improvement (IHI) expressed a little surprise when I said I'd like to run the IHI from Anchorage for a year. It wasn't exactly part of our strategic plan. But after a short, respectful period of hysterical laughter they said, "Go for it," or something colorful with the same gist.

My staff was quite supportive. They gave me earmuffs, several copies of "The Cremation of Sam McGee," and melatonin. They wrote a song called "Yukon Don." I was actually prepared for a culture shock. I was briefly reassured on my first hike in Anchorage when this bearded guy passed me wearing a T-shirt that said on the front, "Earth First." "Okay," I thought to myself. "There are liberal politics out here just like in Boston. But then I read the back of his shirt as he passed me. It said, "We'll log the other planets later."

The women in the audience may get a bit of a kick out of a repeating experience my wife had as she yanked our family, kicking and screaming, into this adventure. Maybe thirty or forty times since it all started people have come up to her and said something like, "You moved to Alaska. Why? Did Don get a job offer there?" Or worse, "That Don Berwick, he's so ready to try anything!" And all the time she's trying to pry my fingers off the banister in our house in Boston.

Anyway, it has begun to work out really well. It's beautiful territory and we've fallen in love with it.

About 217 years before Ann, an innovator, chose Alaska for a change, another person was on his way to Anchorage too. His name was James Cook, a British navy captain, and I want to spend a few minutes talking with you about him.

We have a little game in our family. Every now and then we ask a person at the dinner table, "Who in the history of the world is the one person you would most like to meet and spend an hour talking with?" My experience with my family is that the preferences change over time. My son, Ben, is now in his second year at Harvard, and his favorite historical figure to meet has just changed from Roger Clemens to Alexis de Toqueville, which I think is progress. Dan, his eighteen-year-old brother, has been sticking with Attila the Hun for some years for his own reasons. On a national scale, the name that comes up most frequently is Madonna. I could go with that, but I myself think Shakespeare would be kind of cool, or maybe Sir Isaac Newton. But if you really make it real for me, the person who keeps popping to mind is Captain James Cook—not Kirk, Cook— and he blows my mind.

To understand James Cook, you have to look at a map of the whole world. Here is a person, a little like my wife, who was unable to allow the boundaries of assumption and familiarity to shape his life and his times. During his three key voyages of discovery, from 1768 through 1780, in an era when a trip from London to Bristol could take days, Cook made the whole Earth his playground.

Simply to show where Cook went, you have to show a map of the entire world. I show this to my family when they complain about my travel schedule. Cook proved that New Zealand had two islands. He was the first person to map the eastern coast of Australia, as well as the St. Lawrence River estuary. He went around the Cape of Good Hope four times and Cape Horn twice. He visited Kamchatka, Russia; Japan; Macao, China; and modern Indonesia, and he came within thirty-five miles of Antarctica. He also explored the coast of Alaska, right through the Bering Straits, and almost as far north as the northernmost point, Barrow.

And he did all of that in a small wooden ship, barely one hundred feet long and twenty-nine feet wide, with a crew averaging ninety-five people, most of whom drank heavily and were under twenty-five years of age. When the bottom of his first ship, the *Endeavour*, was ripped open on the Great Barrier Reef, which he discovered in one of the great "oops" of the eighteenth century, Cook sailed the leaking, sinking boat for six more days. He beached it on a barren Australian shore and turned it on its side. He constructed a small village from scratch in the wilderness, and he rebuilt the ship's bottom, plank by plank, in six weeks, before he continued his voyage of twelve months and twelve thousand miles back to England.

And you are complaining about making your merger work!

But Cook wasn't just a superb sailor. He was also a first-rate scientist and a terrific manager. He innovated constantly. He tested new clocks for measuring longitude, and new telescopes for navigation and astronomy. His personal observations of the transit of Venus were some of the best in the world. His surveys of the St. Lawrence River were the most reliable for over a century. And he beat scurvy.[1]

This scurvy story deserves a bit of a detour—as if this whole speech doesn't seem to be a detour so far—because it has a lot to do with my main topic, which I haven't gotten to yet—namely, the spread of innovation.

For many centuries, scurvy was the main threat to the health of naval crews. When Vasco da Gama sailed around the Cape of Good Hope for the first time in 1497, 100 of his crew of 160 men died of scurvy. Cook, by contrast, lost only three men to that disease in his three voyages. Nobody knew about vitamin C at that time, but some dietary factor was suspected. Captain James Lancaster proved it in 1601. In that year, commanding a fleet of four ships on a voyage from England to India, Lancaster gave the crew on one ship three teaspoons of lemon juice every day. At the halfway point on the trip, 110 out of 278—40 percent—of the sailors on the three other ships had died of scurvy, but none had died on the ship with the lemon juice.[2]

No one seemed to notice, however; despite Lancaster's evidence, practices in the Royal Navy did not change. The study was repeated 146 years later, in 1747, by a British navy physician named James

Lind. In a random trial of six treatments for scorbutic sailors on the HMS *Salisbury*, citrus again proved effective against scurvy; victims largely recovered in a matter of a few days.[3] It still took the Royal Navy 48 more years to react and at last order that citrus fruits be a part of the diet on all navy ships. Scurvy in the Royal Navy disappeared almost overnight. The British Board of Trade took seventy more years to adopt the innovation, ordering proper diets on merchant marine vessels in 1865. The total time elapsed from Lancaster's definitive study to universal British preventive policy on scurvy was 264 years.

The problem of scurvy obsessed Captain James Cook. He did not focus on citrus as the cure (a mistake that actually delayed navy action), but on a combination of good hygiene and sauerkraut, which also contains quite a bit of vitamin C. For reasons that anyone who has eaten sauerkraut in close quarters can understand, the sailors under Cook resisted these dietary orders, but Cook made it his business to ensure deployment of sauerkraut in the diets of everyone on his voyages and even once flogged a sailor for refusing to eat his sauerkraut. More important, Cook ordered his officers to eat it also, writing in his journal words that all senior executives should have emblazoned in their minds: "To introduce any new article of food among seamen, let it be ever so much for their good, requires both the examples and the authority of a Commander."

The Slow Pace of Spreading Change in Health Care

When it comes to health care innovation, many health care executives and clinical leaders seem to lack Cook's success in getting people to "eat the sauerkraut." Their organizations and staff act more like the Royal Navy than like James Cook and his crew. Even when an evidence-based innovation is implemented successfully in one part of a hospital or clinic, it may spread slowly or not at all to other parts of the organization.

The problem of the slow spread of change applies not only to sound, formally studied, bioscientific innovations, such as appear in medical journals, but also to the numerous effective process innovations that arise from improvement projects of our own latter-day Lancasters and Linds in local settings, pilot sites, and progressive organizations. In health care, invention is hard, but spread seems even harder.

In recent projects sponsored by the IHI and in other published studies, for example, the following frustrating circumstances have surfaced. A few pioneering obstetricians and nurses in a community hospital were able to safely reduce their cesarean section rates from 26 percent to 15 percent, but rates remained high for most of the other obstetricians in the hospital.[4] A large HMO supported a benchmark asthma program in one medical center, with hospitalization rates down by two-thirds and drug-prescribing practices nearly totally consistent with the best national recommendations, but the rest of the medical centers in the HMO continued unaffected.[5] In a multihospital system, the general surgeons at one hospital agreed to standardize suture materials, stapling devices, and surgical tray setups, saving the hospital millions of dollars and reducing errors dramatically, but surgeons in the other system hospitals fought standardization tooth and nail.[6] Randomized trials have shown that simple, cheap antibiotics are best for first ear infections in children, yet in a study of twelve thousand children with first ear infections in the Colorado Medicaid program, 30 percent received unnecessary, expensive, and hazardous antibiotics, at an excess cost of more than $200,000 per year.[7]

I could go on, but you get my point.

On a more general level, the pattern is actually a little more complicated. I call it "The Three Bears" of the spread of innovation: too slow, too fast, and just right.

I just offered you some examples of too slow: innovations that are ready for prime time, that are backed by plenty of evidence but just don't spread—such as lemon juice for scurvy. Here are some other, current examples: treating asthma with anti-inflammatory agents instead of bronchodilators, using breast-conserving surgery for certain stages of breast cancer, emphasizing patient involvement in decision making, substituting inexpensive for expensive antibiotics, using basic queuing theory to reduce waiting times. All of these are changes that have spread much too slowly for our own good.

Sometimes, though, changes spread too fast, and that causes a different kind of damage. Some drugs enter common use much faster than their advantage merits. Much of the otitis media in this country is treated with inappropriate broad-spectrum antibiotics. Augmentin is not the drug of first choice for otitis, but it is commonly used that way, and such use began within a few months of its licensing.

The U.S. Preventive Services Task Force, of which I was vice chair, reviewed preventive and screening technologies and found many that were growing rapidly in use without any scientific proof of their merit—and often with some proof of their harm. These include techniques such as continuous monitoring for preterm labor, prostatic ultrasound tests, and exercise stress testing in normal adults to screen for coronary disease. I think the current wave of acquisition of physician practices as a corporate strategy may fit in this category of too fast as well. There isn't any real proof that it's a great strategy, and there is lots of evidence that it's an expensive one.

There are also some tantalizing examples of what I would call "just right" spread. One recent, dramatic example is immunization against Hemophilus influenzae B, which was one of the most common causes of bacterial meningitis in children when I was in training but now is almost gone. The following graph shows the trajectory of this disease over the past decade, which matches perfectly the deployment of a safe, effective vaccine (Figure 5.1). As soon as the knowledge was ready, we put it to use and beat this disease almost completely.

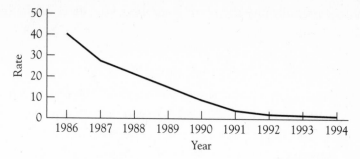

Figure 5.1. Incidence of Hemophilus Influenzae B, 1986–1994.
Source: Centers for Disease Control, "Progress Toward the Elimination of Hemophilus Influenzae Type B Disease Among Infants and Children." *Morbidity and Mortality Weekly Report*, October 25, 1996, 45(42), 901–906.

Here is the lesson: generating good changes is not the same as putting those good changes to use. The problems of creating innovation and using innovation overlap, but they are not the same. Mama Bear and Papa Bear, too fast and too slow, still win.

The Science of Diffusion of Innovation

I have been studying this problem for a while now and have come across not just a little help but a lot. It turns out that an enormous body of research exists to help us understand this sauerkraut problem. Let me review it briefly.

The study of diffusion of innovation has a long and deep history in social science, with important modern contributions by Everett Rogers (especially his landmark text, *Diffusion of Innovations*[8]), Andrew Van de Ven (especially his leadership of the Minnesota Innovation Research Program[9]), and many others. These students of the spread of innovation focus on three basic clusters of influence that, in descriptive studies, correlate with the rate of spread of a change: (a) *perceptions of the innovation;* (b) *characteristics of the people who adopt the innovation,* or fail to do so; and (c) *contextual factors*, especially involving communication, incentives, leadership, and management.

Perceptions of the Innovation

Perceptions of an innovation predict between 49 and 87 percent of the variance in the rate of spread.[10] In particular, five perceptions, or properties of the change as possible adopters understand it, seem most influential.

First, and most powerful, is the *perceived benefit* of the change. People are more likely to adopt an innovation if they think it can help them. This is a more complicated idea than it appears, however, because for most people who accept or reject an innovation, *benefit* is a relative matter—a matter of the balance between risks and gains, and of risk aversion in comparing the known status quo (without the innovation) with the unknown future (if the innovation is adopted). The relevant calculation of value involves risk and benefit. The more knowledge individuals can gain about the expected consequences of an innovation—leading to what Rogers calls "reduction in uncertainty"—the more likely they will be to adopt it.[11] Most people are not like James Cook; they do not go looking for trouble and calling it "adventure." They go looking for ways to stay out of trouble, especially unfamiliar trouble. They tend, therefore, to avoid novelty, and unfamiliar changes bear an extra burden of proof.

Why is a difficult question. One of my colleagues found this quote from Montaigne, which may help: "The legislator of the Thurians ordained that whosoever would go about either to abolish an old law or to establish a new should present himself with a halter about his neck to the people, to the end that if the innovation he would introduce should not be approved by everyone, he might immediately be hanged."

Second, to diffuse rapidly, an innovation must be *compatible* with the values, beliefs, history, and current needs of people. For example, only a minority of physician groups routinely use formal, scientific protocols and guidelines in their practices.[12] This may be due in part to stubbornness, but it may also involve the guidelines' lack of compatibility with current processes. Even a scientifically reasonable guideline may simply not work well in the current context. In addition, to spread quickly, a change must resonate with currently felt needs and belief systems. Surgeons do not become interested in finding new ways to arrive in the operating room on time if they do not care when the surgery starts or if they "know" that the reason surgeons show up late is because operations do not start on time, instead of *vice versa*. Obstetricians do not become interested in exploring ways to reduce cesarean section rates if they believe that current rates are clinically acceptable or necessary to avoid malpractice suits.

A third factor affecting the rate of diffusion is the simplicity of the proposed innovation. Generally, simple innovations spread faster than complicated ones. Individuals who develop an innovation are often not its best salespeople, because they are usually at least as invested in its complexity as in its elegance. They tend to insist on absolute replication, not adaptation. However, innovations are more robust in the face of modification than their inventors think, and local adaptation, which often involves simplification, is nearly a universal property of successful spread. In fact, the Minnesota Innovation Research Program found that innovations *always* change as they spread.[13] In a successful diffusion process, the original innovation itself mutates into many different but related innovations.

The word *spread* is a misnomer; a better word is *reinvention*. The way children learn language is a good analogy.[14] The process of language acquisition is much more than copying; it involves interactions between children's brains and the words they hear. In fact, children who only repeat what they hear are not good learners; they are autistic. Individuals in organizations are not autistic; they are learners. They do not just repeat what they hear; they change it. This universal reinvention process may be related to Gerald Nadler's insufficiently famous "uniqueness principle," which states, "No two problems are the same."[15] Neither are any two solutions.

One common adaptation is to simplify the change. A successful clinical improvement project at Intermountain Health Care's LDS Hospital, led by Carol Ashton, reduced the rate of pressure sores in vulnerable patients by 80 percent or more through the "adoption" of one of the clinical guidelines published by the Agency for Heath Care Policy and Research.[16] I will always remember Carol's comment when I grilled her about how this was accomplished; she reflected that she and her colleagues had actually "adopted" the guidelines only in the most general sense of the word. They found that the thirty-page guideline book contained two changes with especially high leverage: calculate a decubitus ulcer risk score via the Braden Scale,[17] and turn high-risk patients every two hours. These two simple innovations, not the whole detailed, complex guideline, however scientific its pedigree, produced the lion's share of the result. In fact, it seems fair to say that the Intermountain team actually *failed* to adopt the guideline; instead, they reinvented their own locally adapted version of the innovation and put it to work.

Two other perceptions predict the spread of an innovation: *trialability* (whether or not a proposed adopter believes he or she can figure out a way to test the change on a small scale without implementing it everywhere at first) and *observability* (the ease with which potential adopters can watch others try the change first).

Changes spread faster when they have these five perceived attributes: benefit, compatibility, simplicity, trialability, and observability.

Characteristics of the People Who Adopt the Innovation

A second cluster of factors that helps explain the rate of spread of an innovation is that associated with the personalities of the people among whom spread might occur—the potential "adopters." The prevailing model of population stratification comes originally from a 1943 study of the rate of adoption of a new form of hybrid seed corn among Iowa farmers (Figure 5.2).[18,19] In some ways the

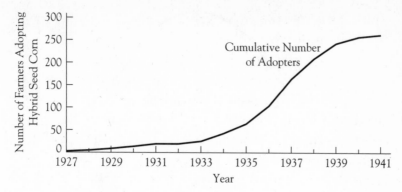

Figure 5.2. Number of Adopters of Hybrid Seed Corn in Two Iowa Communities.

Source: Rogers, E. M., *Diffusion of Innovations*, 4th ed. (New York: Free Press, 1995). Reprinted with permission of The Free Press, a Division of Simon & Schuster Adult Publishing Group. Copyright © 1995 by Everett M. Rogers. Copyright © 1962, 1971, 1983 by The Free Press.

granddaddy of empirical studies of diffusion, this Iowa study has been replicated since for numerous other innovations. Its authors found that the curve of adoption of the innovation among three hundred farmers had an S-shape, with an early slow phase affecting very few farmers, a rapid middle phase with a wide spread, and a slow third phase with incomplete penetration in the end. It looks much like the epidemic curve of a contagious disease.

Over time, students of innovation came to classify the underlying population of adopters into five categories (Figure 5.3). Because these categories were defined statistically, based simply on the number of standard deviations from the median adoption time, the classification is somewhat artificial. Nonetheless, the resulting labels have entered conventional use and have proven helpful as a model of variation in adoption behaviors.

The fastest adopting group (by definition, two standard deviations or more faster than the mean rate of adoption, and therefore, by definition, about 2.5 percent of those involved) is called *Innovators*. They are distinguished from the rest of the population by their venturesomeness, tolerance of risk, fascination with novelty, and

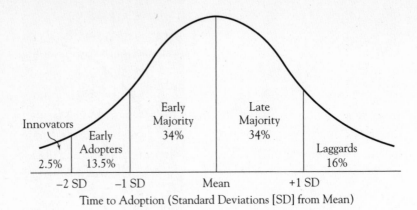

Figure 5.3. Adopter Categorization on the Basis of Innovativeness.

Source: Rogers, E. M., *Diffusion of Innovations,* 4th ed. (New York: Free Press, 1995). Reprinted with permission of the Free Press, a Division of Simon & Schuster Adult Publishing Group. Copyright © 1995 by Everett M. Rogers. Copyright © 1962, 1971, 1983 by The Free Press.

willingness to "leave the village" to learn, as it were. Rogers calls them *cosmopolite*.[20] They belong to cliques that transcend geographical boundaries, and they invest energy in those remote connections. Innovators who were studied in traditional Colombian villages left on trips to cities about 30 times a year, while the average resident left 0.3 times a year.[21] Innovators tend to be wealthier than average or to have special circumstances that give them enough slack to accept the risks inherent in innovating. Locally, they tend to be a little socially disconnected. They are not opinion leaders; in fact, they may be thought of as weird or incautious. In health care, physician-innovators may be thought of as mavericks or may appear to be heavily invested personally in a specialized topic.

The next group, called *Early Adopters* (by definition between one and two standard deviations quicker to adopt than the average, and therefore about 13 percent of people) are different from Innovators. They are opinion leaders; they are locally well-connected socially, and they do not tend to search quite so widely as the Innovators. They do, however, make it a point to talk with Innovators and with one another. They cross-pollinate and they select ideas that they would like to try out. They have the resources and the risk tolerance to try new things. Such people are generally testing several innovations at once and can report on them if asked. They are self-conscious experimenters. Most crucial to the dynamics of spread, Early Adopters are watched. In health care settings they are probably often chosen as elected leaders or representatives of a clinical group, and they are the likeliest targets of pharmaceutical company detailing.

The people who watch the Early Adopters, the next third of the distribution, are the *Early Majority*. Whereas the Early Adopters maintain bridges to the outside through Innovators, often by traveling, actually or virtually, the Early Majority are quite local in their perspectives. They learn mainly from people they know well and they require personal familiarity and trust—more than trust in science or theory—before they test a change. They may be somewhat less well-endowed with resources than the first two groups, and therefore less able to take risks. Those in the Early Majority are readier to hear about innovations relevant to current, local problems than to hear about general "background" improvements. (Dairy farmers are more ready to accept innovations in dairy farming than in general animal care.) Physicians in the Early Majority are more ready to try those innovations that meet their immediate needs than to try those that are simply interesting ideas.

The next group, another third of the population, is even more conservative: the *Late Majority*. While the Early Majority look to the Early Adopters for signals about what is safe to try, the Late Majority look to the Early Majority for such signals. They will adopt an innovation when it appears to be the new status quo (for physicians, the standard of practice), not before. They watch for local proof; they do not find remote, cosmopolite sources of knowledge to be either trustworthy or particularly interesting.

Members of the final group are sometimes called *Laggards*; they are the 16 percent of the people for whom, in Rogers' term, "the point of reference . . . is the past."[22] The term *laggards* probably misstates this group's value and wisdom. They should perhaps be called traditionalists, sea anchors, or archivists, to emphasize that they often make choices that are wise and useful to the community or organization. Some never change, and thank goodness, because they help us remember where we came from. They are the physicians who swear by the tried and true.

Contextual Factors

A third cluster of factors influencing the rate of diffusion of innovations are contextual and managerial factors within an organization or social system that encourage and support, or discourage and impede, the actual processes of spread. For example, organizations may be nurturing environments for Innovators, offering them encouragement, resources, and security for their inevitable failures, or they may discourage Innovators by asking all employees not to rock the boat and by regarding those who propose change as troublemakers. Similarly, because the Early Majority tends to learn about innovations best from local and social interactions with Early Adopters, organizations that foster such social exchanges may see faster spread of changes than organizations that develop habits of isolation or whose buildings have architectural features that discourage hallway chats.

Rogers also points out that leaders have several styles of spread and make "innovation-decisions" of three types: *optional, collective,* and *authority*.[23] No one style is best in all circumstances or for all innovations. (I failed to adopt a new, superior word-processing program until my officer manager one night erased the old one from my computer and threw out all existing copies of it that were in the office. This authority maneuver spread the change into my work in a single day, whereas the optional spread strategy had failed for a year.) The managerial task, and art, is to fit the strategy to the change and to the social context. By the same token, organizations with an impoverished stylistic repertoire—for example, always using authoritarian approaches or always seeking consensus before acting—may be puzzled that some changes spread quickly, while others don't spread at all.

The Dynamics of Diffusion

The curve that describes the spread of innovation has a tipping point, after which it becomes difficult to stop a change from spreading further. Changes appear to acquire their own momentum in this way somewhere on the ascending portion of the adoption curve, often between 15 percent and 20 percent adoption.[24] This empirical finding makes theoretical sense in view of the social dynamics in the population model of adoption. Once Innovators and Early Adopters (about 15 percent of the population) have embraced a change, the model asserts, the Early Majority will follow their lead (if they can interact with them); and once the Early Majority have done so, the Late Majority will discover that the majority has changed direction and will feel comfortable changing too.

This dynamic implies that successful diffusion depends more on how an organization or social system deals with its Innovators, Early Adopters, and the interface between Early Adopters and the Early Majority than with any other groups or phases.

This literature on diffusion of innovation is a little dry, and it tends to be descriptive, not prescriptive. I would like to give you some educated guesses about how we can get better at helping innovations to spread, and at slowing down the ones that shouldn't. To get help in this, I'd like to introduce you to another innovation expert, beyond my wife and Captain Cook, and have her tell you her own story. Her name is Eleanor McMullen, and the tape you're about to see was made in 1990 by some high school students in her hometown of Port Graham, Alaska. The tape's technical quality is poor, but it's worth listening carefully for Mrs. McMullen's lessons. She is a master of change and she knows, I think, what she's talking about. I also think you have lots of Eleanor McMullens in your organizations, and maybe listening to her will help you think about how to help them.

Eleanor McMullen and James Cook have something in common, by the way. When Captain Cook came to Alaska and took a right turn on May 28, 1778, up what would later be called Cook Inlet, ending where Anchorage sits today, his ship, the *Resolution*, passed the homes of Eleanor McMullen's ancestors. They were probably there, the Eyak Indians, watching the *Resolution* sail past their barren beaches at what is now called the town of Port Graham, Alaska, population 179. Two hundred years later, Eleanor McMullen would be on her own journey right there, in Port Graham, covering only a few miles, not Cook's tens of thousands, but using every bit of Cook's courage and ingenuity as a leader of exploration, innovation, and systemic change. Let me begin by letting Mrs. McMullen establish her credentials. *[At this point in the speech, Dr. Berwick plays a series of video clips from an interview with Eleanor McMullen.]*

> *Video Clip 1.* First of all, my mother was an Alaskan native, born and raised in this area. But she was an alcoholic also. Both my parents are deceased. My father was nonnative, was not into substance or alcohol abuse, but was a victim of my mother's alcohol abuse. I came from a family of seven children. Three children died as infants or toddlers and there were four of us that grew up, a brother and three of us girls. Of the four that grew up, two were severely into alcohol almost all their adult lives and one sister was occasionally an alcoholic, and I had one sister that was a victim of sexual abuse. So we have a wide range of things we had to grow up with in our family. I'm a mother of five children, grandmother to six children, and in my family I have a son who's a recovering alcoholic. I have a husband who's a recovering alcoholic. We know what alcohol is and sexual abuse and how they can affect our lives. So it caused a lot of confusion, a lot of confusion in thinking of who I was and what I could be and how could I do anything because I

was so good for nothing. I just want to make sure everybody knows that I know what I'm talking about—the pain of a child growing up.

At first, in her adolescent dawn, Mrs. McMullen believed the message that she was worthless, and she planned her own suicide. A brother rescued her. He took her to his cabin and drew masks for her, asking her to wear them in front of a mirror and then choose between the masks and her own face. She chose her own face, and that was a turning point. Change agents often have a deep understanding of the system they wish to change.

Mrs. McMullen left Port Graham, married, and moved to Iowa—where the seed corn studies had been done—and lived there for seven years. Then, hearing that her parents were ill, she decided to return to Port Graham, where she lives today. That was twenty years ago. When she went back, with her new, cosmopolite eyes, and through the eyes of her new young children, she saw her home differently. People who lead change must usually leave their current environment in order to grasp what others cannot see. Listen as Mrs. McMullen describes her new viewpoint, and then listen to the reactions she encountered.

> *Video Clip 2.* There were three or four of us people that got together and we were going to bring about change in Port Graham. We invited Dr. Richards from ANMC [Alaska Native Medical Center] and we decided we were going to find a cure for Port Graham. Inviting him, we thought maybe we could find a way to solve the problem of alcoholism. We discovered through what he had to say to us that there were no cures for the alcoholism. We had to do something as a community about it. He could find and make referrals to us on how we could go about making ordinances and bringing about voting the community dry. When our local villagers found out about the

discussion that we had with Dr. Richards we were verbally harassed. We were cursed. We were put down. People didn't want the village to be dry. They didn't want control over the alcohol brought in. We were practically run out of the community. Those people that verbally harassed us about the meeting we had with Dr. Richards were native and nonnative. In 1975 I approached the village council, after meeting with Dr. Richards about what services could we get into the village and what kinds of programs could we get to help our people sober up. The village council at that time had no answers but referred me to many outside services and said maybe these people can provide answers and suggestions. We didn't get a whole lot of support at that time from the village council. In fact, we were ridiculed.

"In fact, we were ridiculed." I can only imagine what it was like for a woman in a town of 179 people to experience this level of rejection and potential ostracism. I wonder if would-be agents of change in our own organizations may experience similar discomfort or even pain.

She says, "I was ridiculed." But she didn't stop. Effective change agents, like my wife with me, don't take no for an answer. They exhibit a kind of doggedness that I can only call courage. Like lots of innovators, Mrs. McMullen sought support outside the current system and began to recruit inside as well. And Mrs. McMullen focused first on *herself*.

Video Clip 3. Most of all, I think the biggest message that we made available to our community was the fact that we were not going to tolerate violence. We passed that message to our men and to the people in our community because large proportions of those people were men that were doing the physical and sexual violence against other people. And we were giving a message that we were not going to tolerate—we were not going to put up with such a thing, and that people and women were going to have choices and were making those choices. Slowly I realized I myself needed change, needed lots of work. Through all the exposure that I had, one of the very first programs I was exposed to was the "Here's Looking at You" program. I went to Anchorage for a one-day workshop and training so I could bring it back to my village and provide training in the school system. It was difficult for me to even negotiate with the principal and the school at the time to provide me time, one hour a day, to work with the kids. The other thing was, the community's acceptance of the program itself was difficult. I had to do a lot of PR. I have the highest regard for two people that I think really promoted and brought about change in my region. Without them, I feel like we would never have gotten a lot of programs off the ground. They're the people that talked about the issues when nobody else was willing to talk about them, who were willing to deal with those issues and educate the people in the communities that provided the services. One of the really important things that I think they did was to plant seeds. When I go to school or when I learn something, I don't always keep it just bottled up within myself but I share it with people, and I consider that planting seeds. And whatever little seed I have planted somewhere will grow. Sometimes the growth is real slow and then there's a time when it's quite rapid.

Planting seeds. Everett Rogers says that Innovators are not often well-connected socially. They have outside connections that are strong, but inside ones are weakened by the threat of change they bring with them. It takes a long time for a change agent to build momentum, to shift from the change agent role to the Early Adopter role. At this point, you see changes becoming an "inside job." It is very, very hard work. I love the names of Captain Cook's ships because they so capture what it took: *Endeavour* and *Resolution*.

> *Video Clip 4.* In order to bring more change into my community, I had to become involved in a lot of health areas and related programs. One of them was the interim mental health board. I served in that capacity for nine years. In order to get services into the village, we had to be involved and constantly battle for the dollars and getting people to come into the community. I was really hopeful that immediately sobriety would be occurring in our communities and people would be making a lot of change in their families and lives.

At this point, Mrs. McMullen ran into the problem that change theorists call *reinvention*. I could describe the theory, but she does it better in her own words. It was another turning point.

> *Video Clip 5.* No matter how many services families received, or how much counseling individuals received, we still had a problem. It never seemed to go away or get better. The stressing thing of it all was just because we had a program dealing with alcoholism didn't mean that change was going to occur immediately. We had a counselor we hired and still there was rampant alcoholism. I couldn't understand why there wasn't more sobriety in our communities. Then the realization struck me that we as people had a lot to do with it, and in order to bring about change we had to do something locally in the community. We could not be expecting someone from the outside to come in and make change.

That was the big thing that we were doing in my community. I was doing. I was thinking that programs that would develop in the lower forty-eight states or develop in Anchorage or in Juneau or someplace else were going to come in and make change in this community. It didn't work. We had to develop our own programs and make our programs work here in the community itself. It couldn't happen if the local people didn't do it. That's what it took to bring about change and there continues to be change in Port Graham only because people are involved.

Now, one of the characteristics of "ownership" that Mrs. McMullen emphasizes is that leading change requires an investment of self. Leaders of change have to change themselves. The next segment on leadership could have been written by Captain Cook himself.

Video Clip 6. Leadership is one of the things I think is very important—that the leadership in a community be sober, be responsible, be nonabusive, be nonjudgmental. I think that person needs to be involved in healing and wellness themselves. That's one of the things that I wholeheartedly support and promote. I'm hoping eventually that all the council members on the village council now have some kind of treatment to help them in their progress. They may not be alcohol users, but they grew up in a village where when one person is drunk, everybody is affected by the drunkenness of that one person. So we've been affected in one way or another in being dysfunctional ourselves and developing survival skills. And in order to help and be a leader in our community, I think that person needs to be a well-healed person.

The biggest threats that the Alaskan native population face today are alcoholism, substance abuse, and violence—exactly as Eleanor McMullen described them in Port Graham. But in Port Graham those threats are now, for the moment, at bay. It is fascinating to me that English Bay, a community only twenty miles from Port Graham, hasn't made anywhere near the progress that Port Graham has against child abuse, suicide, depression, and alcoholism. But at least in Port Graham today, Mrs. McMullen says she knows of only six or seven active alcoholics, alcohol-related motor vehicle injuries have nearly ended, and alcohol-related clinic visits have dropped dramatically.

> *Video Clip 7.* We feel like we need to be in control as a village of our problems that may exist. We need to be involved in them actively and to make recommendations and to follow up and monitor whatever problem that they're involved in. The programs available for treatment are endless, and I hope your organization has been able to gain some information from this in the growth of Port Graham to what it is now. I don't want to paint a rosy picture, but I want to let you know that Port Graham has grown from a violent community to a community now that has so much pride of its children, of its families, of its people, and continues to grow. Thank you.

From Description to Prescription

Let me tell you what I think I have learned from these explorers about leading change. The lessons are not easy ones, especially for me. The world doesn't work the way I—and other impatient people—wish it would. Using knowledge takes a lot more time and energy than gaining knowledge. So I'm going to suggest some rules—Berwick's rules for spreading good change. They're only guesses, courtesy of James Cook of the Royal Navy and Eleanor McMullen of Port Graham, Alaska.

RULE 1: *Find sound innovations.*

This is almost too obvious to say, but too important to leave unsaid. Unlike those in other industries, health care Innovators do tend to publish their work. Professional journals abound with their stories. Yet in many health care organizations, even large ones, no formal mechanisms exist for identifying changes that should be deployed. Few senior management structures in health care arrange for routine, high-level surveillance of even a few scientific journals for ideas that should be spread. Instead, senior leaders seem to leave this process to an imagined, latent professional culture that they assume is constantly scanning for new ideas. Unfortunately, that culture, at a system level, does not do such combing.[25,26] Medical communities, like most other communities, are primarily local in their orientation, are dominated numerically by Early and Late Majority groups, and do not trust remote and personally unfamiliar sources of authority. (Eleanor McMullen would be no more welcome in most health care organizations than she was at first in Port Graham.) The counterweight ought to be a formal system of search for innovations. Health care organizations need to manage the interface between the organization and scientific knowledge more deliberately than they currently do.[27]

RULE 2: *Find and support Innovators.*

People who search for innovations are crucial to our future. Basic answers to chronic, local problems tend to come from outside the current system. Those who mean to manage change as senior leaders should identify and value these scouts and should give them the slack and resources to look in distant places. Innovators will not be the easiest people to deal with in the organization; they may be abrasive, not invested in local networks, and demanding of latitude. If they were not, they would not be Innovators. In this regard, it may help to know that in a review of sixty-one major inventions since the year 1900, forty (two thirds) came from individuals act-ing alone, not from corporate research and development efforts.[28] The village council didn't like what it heard from Eleanor McMullen; they saw her as a troublemaker. Innovators are dia-monds in the rough.

RULE 3: *Invest in Early Adopters*.

Leaders may decrease resistance to the spread of innovation if they stop concentrating management attention on compliance by everyone and start investing heavily in the curiosity of a few Early Adopters. This switch from compliance to support is crucial to effective diffusion. It is equally important to know who the poten-tial Early Adopters are. Like Innovators, they need the slack time and resources to try out new things and to reduce their uncertainty through small-scale trials. Early Adopters get their news from Inno-vators. Some diffusion researchers call this factor "the strength of weak ties,"[29] emphasizing the value of relatively nonlocal, socially weak relationships in supplying Early Adopters with ideas they can play with. Leaders who want to accelerate change should help increase the ease and frequency with which Early Adopters meet and interact with Innovators.

RULE 4: *Make Early Adopter activity observable*.

The Early Majority watch the Early Adopters, but they cannot watch them if they cannot see them. The communication channels that work well between these groups are not "media" channels; they are social channels. One cannot effectively support the crucial interface between the Early Adopters and the Early Majority by memoranda or publications. When I asked Eleanor McMullen how her ideas moved from fringe to mainstream in Port Graham, her answer was clear: "Talk. I talked to people. I never stopped talking." This is the same answer I got from Robert DeMott, an Early

Adopter obstetrician in Green Bay, Wisconsin, who helped lead that community's cesarean section rates down from 18 percent to 8 percent.[30] When I asked Bob what he did that mattered most, he said, "Talking to people—to every single obstetrician one-on-one—addressing their questions."

This is, by the way, exactly the answer researchers find when they try to explain the great success of one of the most successful innovation-spread programs ever seen in this country—the Agricultural Extension Service (AES).[31] Moving knowledge to the farmer for use, the AES relies heavily on an extension apparatus of closely integrated tiers, on reducing the social distance at each interface, and more and more on local, face-to-face networks as they move information out into the field. The AES refers to the notion of "a spannable social distance" throughout the chain, ensuring that at every stage between the university and the field, each person hears "the news" from someone socially familiar enough to be credible. Closer to medicine, the pharmaceutical industry has long recognized the power of one-on-one "detailing" of new drugs to doctors and, consequently, continues to invest huge resources in this method of spreading its pharmacological innovations. American health care could benefit greatly from the establishment by the federal government of a health care extension service modeled on the AES.

RULE 5: *Trust and enable reinvention.*

Yogi Berra said, "If you can't imitate him, don't copy him." That is the heart of Nadler's uniqueness principle,[32] and the sound reasoning behind reinvention as a universal process. In innovation, new *concepts* must usually come from outside the current system, but new *processes*—the things that make the concepts work—must come from inside the current system or they will not work. To work, changes must be not only adopted locally but also adapted locally. Many leaders seem to regard this process of reinvention as a form of waste, narcissism, or resistance. It is often none of these. Reinvention is a form of learning and, in its own way, an act of both courage and creativity. It also takes time and energy. I asked Eleanor McMullen about this, because Captain Cook is unavailable, and she said, "Tell those people"—meaning you—"that improving is like peeling an onion. Each change idea leads to many new layers and more ideas. I never could have known at the start where we would be now, and the process never stops." As Van de Ven and his Minnesota research team wrote, "An initial idea tends to proliferate into several divergent and parallel ideas during the innovation process."[33]

RULE 6: *Create slack for change.*

Van de Ven places this idea at or near the top of his priority list for diffusion.[34] In every stratum of adopter, from Innovators to Laggards, a recurrent theme is that adoption takes energy. The Innovators need the energy for cosmopolite search and tinkering; the Early Adopters need the energy to find Innovators and to test promising discoveries; the Early Majority need the energy to network with the Early Adopters, to learn some details of the new way, and to assess risks and benefits; the Late Majority need energy and information to monitor the ambient culture; and the Laggards must have the emotional energy to remain in custody of the past without feeling devalued or too far out of step. These are investments. In real organizations, they involve real time and real money. No system trapped in the continuous throes of production, existing always at the margin of resources, innovates well unless its survival is also imminently and vividly at stake. Even then, leaders who want innovation to spread must make sure they have invested people's time and energy in it.

RULE 7: *Lead by example.*

Leaders who champion the spread of innovation must be prepared for resistance, even ridicule; most important, they must be prepared to begin change with themselves. James Cook had to eat his own sauerkraut, and health care leaders who want to spread change must change themselves first.

Exploration and leading innovation have their pleasures and their risks. They have no shortcuts. The spirit of the people with whom we work and live is the greatest source of untapped energy in our society, but the processes of innovation and spread have their own rules, their own pace, and their own multilayered forms of search and imagining. The pace of change, writes Dr. Joseph Juran, is "majestic."[35] To create a future different from its past, health care needs leaders who understand innovation and how it spreads, who respect the diversity in change itself, and who, drawing on the best of social science for guidance, can nurture innovation in all its rich and many costumes.

Notes

1. Lind, J. *A Treatise of the Scurvy*. Edinburgh: Kincaid and Donaldson, 1753. (Reprinted by Edinburgh University Press, 1953.)

2. Mosteller, F. "Innovation and Evaluation." *Science*, 1981, *211*, 881–886.

3. Lind, *A Treatise of the Scurvy*.

4. Flamm, B., Kabcenell, A., Berwick, D. M., and Roessner, J. *Reducing Cesarean Section Rates While Maintaining Maternal and Infant Outcomes*. Boston: Institute for Healthcare Improvement, 1997.

5. Weiss, K. B., Mendoza, G., Schall, M. W., Berwick, D. M., and Roessner, J. *Improving Asthma Care in Children and Adults*. Boston: Institute for Healthcare Improvement, 1997.

6. Nugent, W. C., Kilo, C. M., Ross, C. S., Marrin, C. A., Berwick, D. M., and Roessner, J. *Improving Outcomes and Reducing Costs in Adult Cardiac Surgery*. Boston: Institute for Healthcare Improvement, 1999.

7. Berman, S., Byrns, P. J., Bondy, J., Smith, P. J., and Lezotte, D. "Otitis Media-Related Antibiotic Prescribing Patterns, Outcomes,

and Expenditures in a Pediatric Medicaid Population." *Pediatrics*, 1997, *100*(4), 585–592.

8. Rogers, E. M. *Diffusion of Innovations* (4th ed.). New York: Free Press, 1995.

9. Schroeder, R. G., Van de Ven, A. H., Scudder, G. D., and Rolley, D. "Managing Innovation and Change Processes: Findings from the Minnesota Innovation Research Program." *Agribusiness Management*, 1986, *2*, 501–523.

10. Rogers, *Diffusion of Innovations*, 206.

11. Rogers, *Diffusion of Innovations*, 168.

12. Casalino, L., Gillies, R. R., Shortell, S. M., and others. "External Incentives, Information Technology, and Organized Processes to Improve Health Care Quality for Chronic Diseases: Results of the First National Survey of Physician Organizations." *JAMA*, 2003, *289*, 434–441.

13. Schroeder, Van de Ven, Scudder, and Rolley, "Managing Innovation and Change Processes," 501–523.

14. Pinker, S. *The Language Instinct: The New Science of Language and Mind*. New York: Morrow, 1994.

15. Nadler, G., and Hibino, S. *Creative Solution Finding: The Triumph of Full-Spectrum Creativity over Conventional Thinking*. Rocklin, Calif.: Prima, 1995.

16. *Pressure Ulcers in Adults: Prediction and Prevention*. Clinical Practice Guideline Number 3. AHCPR Pub. No. 92–0047. Rockville, Md.: Agency for Health Care Policy and Research, May 1992.

17. Bergstrom, N., and Braden, B. J. "Predictive Validity of the Braden Scale Among Black and White Subjects." *Nursing Research*, 2002, *51*, 398–403.

18. Rogers, *Diffusion of Innovations*, 258.

19. Ryan, B., and Gross, N. C. "The Diffusion of Hybrid Seed Corn in Two Iowa Communities." *Rural Sociology*, 1943, 8, 15–24.

20. Rogers, *Diffusion of Innovations*, 299.

21. Rogers, *Diffusion of Innovations*, 274.

22. Rogers, *Diffusion of Innovations*, 265.

23. Rogers, *Diffusion of Innovations*, 372.

24. Rogers, *Diffusion of Innovations*, 259.

25. Covell, D. G., Urman, G. C., and Manning, P. R. "Information Needs in Office Practice: Are They Being Met?" *Annals of Internal Medicine*, 1985, *103*, 596–599.

26. Ely, J. W., Osheroff, J. A., Ebell, M. H., and others. "Obstacles to Answering Doctors' Questions About Patient Care with Evidence: Qualitative Study." *British Medical Journal*, 2002, *324*(7339), 710.

27. Davidoff, F., and Florance, V. "The Informationist: A New Health Profession?" *Annals of Internal Medicine*, 2000, *132*, 996–998.

28. Jewkes, J., Sawaers, D., and Stillerman, R. *The Sources of Invention*. New York: St. Martin's Press, 1958, 72–88.

29. Granovetter, M. "Strength of Weak Ties." *American Journal of Sociology*, 1973, *78*, 1360–1380.

30. DeMott, R. K., and Sandmire, H. F. "The Green Bay Cesarean Section Study I: The Physician Factor as a Determinant of Cesarean Birth Rates." *American Journal of Obstetrics and Gynecology*, 1990, *162*, 1593–1602.

31. Rogers, *Diffusion of Innovations*, 357–364.

32. Nadler and Hibino, *Creative Solution Finding*.

33. Schroeder, Van de Ven, Scudder, and Rolley, "Managing Innovation and Change Processes," 501–523.

34. Schroeder, Van de Ven, Scudder, and Rolley, "Managing Innovation and Change Processes," 501–523.

35. Juran, J. M. *Juran on Quality Improvement*. Leader's manual and participant workbook. Wilton, Conn.: Juran Institute, 1981, 14–17.

. . . .

6

Why the *Vasa* Sank

Commentary

Robert Waller

It should come as no surprise that Donald Berwick's 1997 National Forum keynote speech, "Why the *Vasa* Sank," is a masterpiece of design. He suggests at the outset that perhaps improvement in the health care system is impossible; that perhaps we just need to accept the status quo; that improvement is, after all, overreaching, and because overreaching can be dangerous, maybe we should throw in the towel.

Of course this defeatist tone, while slightly disarming, is short-lived. What follows is the story of why the Swedish warship the *Vasa* sank on its maiden voyage in 1628. Woven into the presentation are the risky adventures of the Berwick family in their trek through the relatively uncharted territory of the Alaskan Brooks Range. Both stories expose the principles—and the pitfalls—of what it means to commit to world-class performance.

Berwick spares no words about the need to commit to world-class health care: "I want to promise our patients and their families things that we have never been able to promise them . . . the guarantees of service, functional outcomes, efficiency, comfort, respect, dignity, and scientific excellence that we have never in history given." He is tired of excuses and wants action . . . *now*.

This keynote speech outlines eight elements necessary to achieve world-class performance: bold aims, improvement as a strategy, the importance of signals and monitors, idealized design, insatiable curiosity, a "continuous dance with the customer," aligning aims with the definition of production, and the commitment to drive out waste. At the end, Berwick adds two more elements necessary for world-class performance: cooperation above all and extreme levels of trust.

This 1997 speech outlines in elegant fashion a blueprint for change, a framework upon which any of us in health care can build our future plans to become world-class performers, no matter what our station might be. The need to do so is more critical and more pressing in 2003 than it was in 1997. Time is moving on. We are all inclined to spend more time than we should "getting ready to get started" on the path to world-class performance.

The date and time to begin the Brooks Range exploration was not to be postponed just because it rained on the day of departure. Neither can we postpone our efforts to move forward with dispatch our improvement agendas in health care. Those we serve, especially our patients, deserve nothing less than our undivided attention to world-class performance . . . now.

Why the *Vasa* Sank

9th Annual National Forum on Quality Improvement in Health Care

Orlando, Florida, December 9, 1997

The great comedian Red Skelton used to have a routine about a character named San Fernando Red and his amazing talking horse. San Fernando Red would show off his horse by asking him, "What's two plus two?" The horse would tap out the answer: "Tap, tap, tap, tap." Red would wait a minute, and then say, "Come on, boy, one more."

That's how I feel a lot when I am meeting with senior management teams in health care these days. They tell me how hard things are, with payers and lawyers nipping at their heels, managed care nipping at their prices, mergers going sour, and physician networks being unproductive. Then I tell them how important it is to improve. Errors are too high, waits are too long, unscientific care is too prevalent, waste is everywhere. They tell me how hard it is out there, and then, like San Fernando Red, I tell them, "Come on, boy, one more."

But somehow I don't think I am making the same mistake as San Fernando Red did. I think I am right about the need for improvement. For every one hundred hospital admissions today, there are seven serious or potentially serious drug errors. That can't be good. Patients everywhere in health care endure waits that would produce riots in restaurants, retail stores, theaters, or even airports. Why should they have to wait so long? As many as 80 percent of hysterectomies are scientifically unnecessary. So are more

Keynote speech presented at the 9th Annual National Forum on Quality Improvement in Health Care, Orlando, Florida, December 9, 1997.

than a quarter of the drugs used for ear infections, most of the ultrasound tests done in normal pregnancies, and almost half of the cesarean sections in the United States. Isn't this, with all due respect, some form of assault and battery, however unintended? We underuse inexpensive medications that could prevent recurrent heart attacks, and overuse expensive tests like MRIs and X-rays for back pain. Across this nation there is a thirty-threefold variation in rate of use of appropriate treatments for early stage breast cancer and a twelvefold variation in prostatectomy rates. And yet, in the midst of all of this waste—perhaps because of it—our medical costs are again rising this year at over twice the rate of inflation. So much could be better.

But maybe improvement is impossible. Maybe we need to accept these gaps between what we know we should do and what we actually do. Let's throw in the towel. Improvement is overreaching, and overreaching can be dangerous. I can prove it. Take the *Vasa* as an example.

The *Vasa*

In 1628, Sweden was an international power. Its empire stretched around most of the Baltic seacoast, and it was becoming deeply involved in what was to be the Thirty Years War. The Swedish king, Gustavus Adolphus II, depended largely on his navy for power. He commissioned the building of three warships, to be the largest and most powerful of their time. Gradually, the construction of the first and grandest of the three, the *Vasa*, became a project of such magnitude that plans for the other two ships were set aside. Building the *Vasa* became Gustavus Adolphus's consuming passion. Its hull was built from a thousand oak trees, it carried sixty-four large guns, it was sixty-nine meters long, its masts were more than fifty meters high, and it was covered with gold leaf and painted sculptures (Figure 6.1).

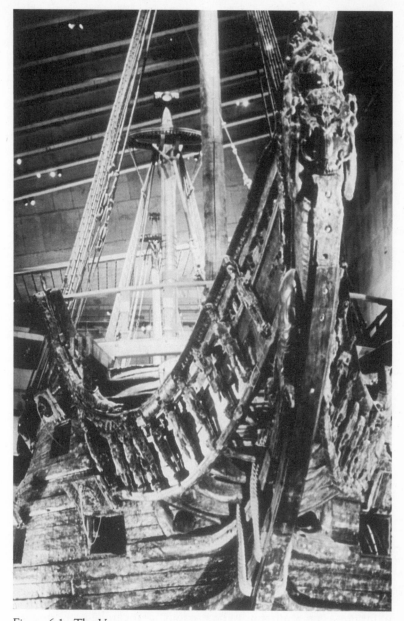

Figure 6.1. The *Vasa*.
   Source: Photo by Hans Hammarskiöld for the *Vasa* Museum, Stockholm,
Sweden.

Gustavus Adolphus searched the world for the best ship designers for the *Vasa,* and he picked a Dutchman, Henrik Hybertson,
as the builder. But the king took a personal interest in the design as
well. He insisted, for example, on an entire extra deck above the
waterline to add to the majesty and comfort of the ship and to make
room for the sixty-four guns he wanted it to carry.

The extra deck also made the ship unstable. The emperor's
innovations went beyond the knowledge base of the shipbuilders
of his time. Several days before the *Vasa* was launched, a stability
test, involving thirty sailors running three times from beam to beam
on the top deck, had to be stopped because the ship was in danger
of capsizing.

Whether or not anyone told the king is uncertain. What is certain is that the *Vasa* was launched on August 10, 1628, in Stockholm harbor in full view of most of the residents of Stockholm, who
had assembled on the wharves for the grand event. The *Vasa* sailed
less than a mile. A gust of wind caught its sails and it tipped vio-
lently to one side, flooded, and sank to the bottom of Stockholm
harbor, where it lay for 333 years, until April 24, 1961, when the
Swedes raised it.

Today the *Vasa* is restored and sits in dry dock at its original construction site. The Swedish have taken the phrase "Every defect is a
treasure" to an impressive extreme and built a major museum
around the *Vasa,* which is now one of the main tourist attractions
in all of Scandinavia.

Silly Gustavus Adolphus. He didn't know when to stop. He
tried to produce a breakthrough, and instead he made a disaster.
Lesson learned.

But wait a minute: What's the lesson here? Not all of our dreams
sink to the bottom of the harbor. Focusing on failure—or the fear
of failure—can remind us to be prudent, or it can be an excuse for
timidity. Let's flip the story for a minute. Let's take a look at success,
and at the kinds of things it takes to keep potential successes from
turning into disasters. I have two case studies for you.

The Brooks Range Trip

Case one: the Berwick family explores the Brooks Range. As you may know, my wife and two of my four children spent the academic year 1996–97 living in Anchorage, Alaska, where my wife had constructed a sabbatical experience as an environmental attorney in the Alaska attorney general's office. My two younger children, Jessica and Becca, and I went along for the ride. As our Alaska swan song in August 1997, we decided to take a two-week trip into the Brooks Range in northern Alaska. We joined another family, making a total party of eleven people: four so-called adults—and seven kids between ten and twenty years of age.

The Brooks Range is wilderness—no fooling. The local national park there, Gates of the Arctic, is, I am told, the only national park in the United States where the Park Service explicitly states as policy that it will not conduct rescues—which is one of the chief criteria my wife used to select it as our destination.

Our plan was to spend eight days hiking 40 miles through the range to the North Fork of the Koyukuk River, where we would meet rafts and a resupply of provisions dropped by plane, and then raft 110 miles in six more days to the outpost bush town of Bettles, Alaska.

It was grueling. "Hiking" in the Brooks Range is a euphemism. It means choosing unmarked routes through trailless terrain, deciding fifty times a day whether to risk walking along a stream drainage where you could get trapped in a gorge or traversing a high slope across slippery tundra toward hidden ravines, or choosing the middle elevations through impenetrable alders. And it rained. We had rain for twelve of our fourteen days on the trail or river, making it a little tough to see the grizzly bears that occasionally wandered a few hundred yards to our left or right, watching us to see if we looked tastier than blueberries.

Preparations for this trip made building the *Vasa* look simple. We packed or flew into the resupply point 420 candy bars, twenty-two rolls of toilet paper, seventeen pounds of granola, twenty-one pounds of angel hair pasta, six pounds of peanut butter, six feet of salami, and three six-person boats. There were 495 person-meals and we used twenty-six U.S. Geological Survey topographic maps.

Not a small project. But we made it—safe and sound. On day 15, our rafts slid gently into Bettles landing, and we celebrated that night with steaks and cherry pie at Bettles Lodge. No *Vasa*, we.

Not long before we left on our Brooks Range trip, another launch took place in Anchorage, and it too went well.

Launching ANMC

Case two is the move of the Alaska Native Medical Center (ANMC) to new digs in Anchorage. ANMC is both the secondary and tertiary care referral hospital for the Alaska Region of the Indian Health Service (IHS) and the main IHS supplier of primary care for the fifty thousand Alaska natives who live in and near the Anchorage bowl. Under IHS guidelines, the old ANMC facility, seriously damaged in the great 1964 Alaska earthquake, had been slated for replacement for many years, and a design and construction project lasting more than five years culminated on June 2, 1997, in a one-day move of all programs, patients, and departments from the old facility in downtown Anchorage to the brand new ANMC about six miles away.

The guiding leaders for the ANMC move were its senior management group, chaired by the CEO—the director in IHS parlance—Dr. Richard Mandsager. I don't know if Dick Mandsager and his colleagues had ever heard about Gustavus Adolphus and the *Vasa*, but I do know they were single-mindedly committed to a successful move from the moment I first heard them speak about it. And they did it. I will try to tell you how they did it. It did not involve timidity.

Committing to World Class

I want to see health care become world class. I want us to promise our patients and their families things that we have never before been able to promise them—the guarantees of service, functional outcomes, efficiency, comfort, respect, dignity, and scientific excellence that we have never in history given. I am not satisfied with what we give them today; like many of you, I am very dissatisfied. And as much respect as I have for the stresses and demoralizing erosion of trust in our industry, I am getting tired of excuses. The theme of this year's National Forum is "Action," and I think we should mean it.

To get there we must become bold. We are never going to get there if timidity guides our aims. Our Brooks Range looms in front of us, and it is called improvement. ANMC moved a hospital, exactly as we must move the performance of our industry. How can we ever do that without sinking our ship? I take that question seriously, and I want to suggest at least some of the elements of "world class," when what we need to accomplish is unprecedented. How to make boldness safe?

The lesson of the *Vasa* does hold. You cannot load more guns and a new deck on the old ship; it will flip over. Marginal aims can be achieved with marginal change, but bold aims require bold changes. The managerial systems and culture that support progress at the world-class level, like the systems and culture that got us through the Brooks Range and that got ANMC moved safely and on time, don't look like business as usual. They are special, and I want to explain them to you. I suggest ten elements of world class, and I'll show you how they appeared in moving a hospital or traversing the mountains. They're not the same as improving, but we can learn from them.

ELEMENT 1: *Bold aims, with tight deadlines*

We will never get where we do not decide to go. Who said, "Cross the Brooks Range"? We did. Who said, "Move the hospital"? The leaders of the IHS and ANMC did. No one told them or us to declare the goal, and both met incredible resistance. It was even harder when we set deadlines. We set out on the Brooks Range trail on August 9. Rain was impending, and it was easy to argue for the 10th, or the 12th, or never. What everyone on that trip knew was fundamental to every successful trek: It must start through an act of pure will. When to take the first step is an arbitrary decision; however, that is not an argument *against*, but the strongest possible argument *in favor of*, setting a start time.

The senior leaders at ANMC set the hospital move date for June 2, 1997, and repeatedly stood firm against proposals to set it back by a week, a month, a couple of months. They knew, maybe intuitively, that the deadline—the arbitrary deadline—would become the most powerful single force they had for organizing the system as a whole. The deadline was not an interpretation of the existing capability; it was an instruction about what capabilities were to be developed. It told people their jobs. Once in place—and once the will of the leaders was tested and found firm—June 2, 1997, became the reference point from which everyone in the system could design their job. Work back from move day and you— each of you—can figure out exactly what you need to be doing, and by when.

To improve now at the pace we ought to, we need bold aims and firm deadlines. Where will our aims come from? Who will declare that we will be error free? That we have a deadline for reducing waits and delays? By when will we stop five hundred thousand unnecessary cesarean sections per year?

When I compare our aims for improvement in health care to those in the world-class companies I saw as a Baldrige judge, nothing impresses me as much as our timidity. Here is our Brooks Range:

- Error-free health care

- Wait-free health care

- Total patient control over decisions

- Evidence-based care, guaranteed

- Costs of care reduced by 30 percent without harm

- A totally revised medical record, with 10 percent decrease in volume and fourfold increase in usefulness

Is this, "Come on, boy, one more"?

Maybe, but world-class organizations don't shy away. They embrace aims like this, and they go at them. That's where Motorola's Six Sigma goals came from, and that's why GE's core strategy is now Six Sigma quality. That's how Roger Milliken decided to take Milliken Corporation to unprecedented cycle times, and how Xerox and Ritz Carlton have committed to 100 percent customer satisfaction. They understand bold aims; we don't yet. With respect to aims, and by comparison to the best in the world, health care is not yet on the map. Let's end that here.

ELEMENT 2: *Improving as the strategy*

Now, at the world-class level, these aims are not merely matters of mission or mantra. They are strategies. Improvement is a strategy. Strategies today in much of health care include merging and, lately, unmerging, downsizing, marketing, pricing, restructuring governance, acquiring physician practices, and developing new sources of capital. That's not what I mean.

Having improvement as a core strategy is not a matter of words. It is a matter of deeds. At the world-class level, strategy, in action, has the regular, even the daily, attention of executives and boards. It involves significant investments of capital and people's time. It is not added on as marginal work. It pushes other work off the plate. By the end of this year GE will have assigned five thousand employees full-time to its Six Sigma efforts. By mid-1998, no one at GE will be promoted who has not completed quality training. That's in a company with just over two hundred thousand employees. They are doing this because of the return on investment. Improvement efforts at GE returned $1.60 for every $1.00 invested in their first year of Six Sigma; next year the return will be 3.5 to 1.

The biggest form of investment is assignment of people. Corporations for which improvement is a strategy define improvement work as productive work. To move successfully, ANMC assigned people both full-time and part-time to managing the move. Marilee White was made a full-time move director. Dr. Richard Brodsky was pulled, at first half-time and then full-time, from his regular job as director of the emergency department to oversee the move of patients from the old site to the new one. Our Brooks Range trip depended on major reallocations of energy—days spent in studying maps, speaking with rangers and guides, acquiring and packing food and equipment.

One special form of assignment—one indicator of serious strategy—is to give special license to people involved centrally in the strategy—I call these "007" assignments. Rules are suspended so that the goal can be achieved. By move day at ANMC, Dr. Brodsky had, in some sense, dictatorial powers. Guided by values, his assignment clear—move patients safely—he was given enormous rope to commandeer resources, bend rules, and create new processes. In the Brooks Range, where difficult decisions came up every hour, it was absolutely necessary to have a leader. We rotated the position, and we never prevented discussion. But the leader's word was the final word, and we agreed to it.

If they are real, strategies get reviewed. The more important the strategy is, the more specific and frequent will be the reviews. At ANMC, the move came to occupy time on absolutely every agenda of internal meeting, including—especially including—the twice-weekly operations meetings of the senior leadership group. I was at no meeting when the move was not discussed. It was like our constantly repeated huddles in the Brooks Range—How far have we come? Where are we on the map? How much water do we have left? How is everyone feeling?

ELEMENT 3: *Signals and monitors*

The aims and the commitment to strategy are not enough. Providing evidence of commitment to aim, giving visible evidence of strategy, is accomplished in part by the management of monitors. Signals evince commitment; strong signals evince strong commitment. Signals are the drumbeat. At ANMC in the months before the move, you could not have been in the building for more than ten seconds without becoming aware that a move was impending. Signs and placards were on every wall and bulletin board. In the main lobby area, and in strategic locations throughout the facility, "countdown" posters were updated every day: "63 days until the move." Newsletters, flyers, and master progress charts were posted in full view of staff and, usually, patients and visitors.

The same was true of the Brooks Range trip. Sacks and resupply barrels were carefully labeled. Our maps were annotated by hand, and we daily marked the position of our camp. Rest stops were announced twenty and ten minutes in advance. The function of such signals was clear—not to pass judgment, but to inform everyone about the state of the system they were part of. It is the exact opposite of the feeling of floating in space that you have when they put you on hold on the telephone. Are they still there? Have I been disconnected? What should I do? Knowing the state of the system you are in is a powerful asset in helping you figure out what to do next. My ten-year-old daughter would have cried if she had no idea when we would rest; but if she knew that the rest stop was coming in ten minutes, she could make plans to hold out.

The science of signals—drumbeats—is called *semiology*. The bolder the goal is, the more crucial semiology becomes. The complex systems in which we work defy visibility. There are no vantage points from which we can easily see the state of the system as a whole. In the Brooks Range, we scouted routes by climbing high on ridges, trying to get a sense of where our local choices were leading us overall. We made marks on maps, triangulated our position over and over again. We weighed and counted food, and interviewed one another about our injuries. We were always trying to make our system visible and to record and learn from our experience and to keep people together.

I call this function *measuring for improvement,* and it has little in common with the familiar forms of measurement in health care today, which I call *measuring for judgment.* Measures for judgment—for selection, approval, reward, punishment, variable compensation—are feared, unwelcome, criticized, and usually gamed. They do *not* illuminate the system—that is not their point. They are indicators of lack of relationship, second-best substitutes for communication when real dialogue is not possible. Measures for improvement have learning as their goal. They are the videotapes we watch after the game to learn from our mistakes. They are the stopwatches of the coaches who help us with our stride. They are what we ask for when we say, "Keep me posted."

At the world-class level, improvement-oriented measures are everywhere: frequent, visible, public, free of blame, frequently reviewed, avidly awaited, and always showing trends over time, because it is over time that we intend to make changes and improve.

ELEMENT 4: *Idealized designs*

Without bold aims, bold improvements never start. Without improvement centered in the resource allocations and visual fields of the strategy-setters of the organization, important improvement cannot continue. Without measurements, the system remains unknown.

But aims, resources, and visible measurements are still not enough. Gustavus Adolphus II found that out pretty well. He did want a big ship, and he put his money where his aim was—he practically ruined the royal treasury. But he forgot about design. After aims, after strategic centering, after measurement comes design.

To understand the importance of design, we need to revisit what I call the First Law of Improvement: *Every system is perfectly designed to achieve exactly the results it gets.* This is a much deeper idea than it may at first appear. It links design and performance—one is just a manifestation of the other. If you want new performance, you're going to have to get yourself a new system.

The following shows a good case study of the linkage between design and performance (Figure 6.2). It's a photo from an old *New England Journal of Medicine* report on an investigation of an outbreak of deaths in a newborn nursery.[1] On the left is a bottle of racemic epinephrine, which is put into the endotracheal tube of babies having trouble breathing. On the right is a bottle of vitamin E, put down the nasogastric tube of premature infants to help them develop. Any guesses about why the babies died? The racemic epinephrine was being put into the nasogastric tube. Any guesses about what happened to the nurses involved in these mishaps? Blamed, of course, for being inattentive or careless—which is stupid. This is a perfectly designed system. It is perfectly designed to kill babies by ensuring a

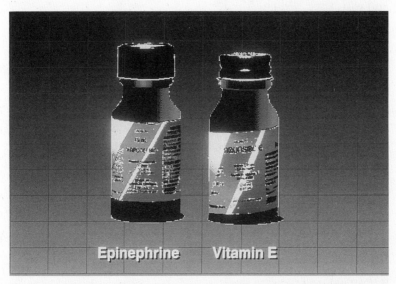

Figure 6.2. Racemic Epinephrine Versus Vitamin E.
Source: New England Journal of Medicine.

specific—low but inevitable—rate of mix-up. Every system is perfectly designed to achieve exactly the results it gets. Get it?

Gustavus Adolphus II put a third deck on a two-deck boat. He didn't design a new system; he stressed an old one. So it sank. You can't just keep asking old processes to accomplish new things; they'll crack.

That's why improvement and change are the same thing. Not all changes are improvements, but all improvements are changes. This is not an easy fact, because we are by nature so committed to the status quo. In fact, we often would rather adhere to the status quo instead of choosing a change with better performance. A couple I know slept over at their friends' house recently and their hosts, insisting that the guest room was uncomfortable, made the guests sleep in the master bedroom while the hosts occupied the guest room. At 2:00 A.M., the hosts' five-year-old son opened the door and wandered into the master bedroom whispering, "Dad? Dad?" The man rolled over and said, "Your dad's not here. He's in the guest room." At which the boy walked around to the other side of the bed and whispered, "Mom? Mom?"

World-class organizations are obsessive in their commitment to world-class designs. They seek changes that can help them. This happens a number of ways, but primarily through the mastery of basic principles of new design. I went over some of these in my Forum speech two years ago, and you may recall my mentioning things like continuous flow, visual controls, standardization, reduction of inspection, and work removal as powerful, modern guiding ideas for new designs with new performance characteristics.

I won't spend my time today on the design concepts themselves. Let me just say that I am now more convinced than ever that organizations that commit to design improvement, as opposed to simply putting new stresses on the current design—more cannon on the same deck—can achieve performance improvement. In the IHI's Breakthrough Series we have now observed and guided almost four hundred teams that spend a year or so together in a topic-specific collaborative to try and knock the socks off performance in designated areas using the most powerful design ideas—change concepts—that science and experts can offer them. About half of the organizations achieve true breakthroughs. When they do invest in proper concepts and proceed rapidly to test changes, they get results. Let me show you some examples—*Vasas* that floated:

- *Reducing waste.* York Hospital in York, Pennsylvania, reduced the inappropriate use of ICU bed days by a physician-nurse team by 90 percent, from 35 percent to fewer than 3 percent, in one year.
- *Using evidence-based care.* A team at Lawrence General Hospital in Lawrence, Massachusetts, reduced cesarean section rates by more than 30 percent in one year, without compromising maternal and infant outcomes. Nash Health Care Systems in Rocky Mount, North Carolina, nearly abolished ventilator-associated pneumonia using protocol-based care. Yale New Haven Hospital's emergency department made significant progress in ensuring scientifically appropriate prescription of oral and inhaled anti-inflammatory agents for emergency room asthma patients.
- *Reducing delays.* Sentara Norfolk Medical Center in Norfolk, Virginia, achieved a 49 percent reduction in postoperative intubation time among coronary surgery patients. St. Joseph's Mercy Hospital in Hot Springs, Arkansas, reduced emergency room waiting time by 50 percent. And Kaiser-Permanente in Sacramento, California, led by Dr. Mark Murray, made substantial reductions in delays in access to office visits.

The ANMC move leaders dealt very carefully with the design of their processes, conducting many small-scale tests of change. By the time move day came, they had engaged in multiple simulations of patient transport, debugging the transportation design each time. They knew that the elevators in the old building frequently broke down, so they reviewed the breakdown logs of the prior three years, learned the failure modes and effects, and created backups and redundancy where they needed it. Our Brooks Range trip required new capabilities in navigation without trails, bear protection, and waterproofing. Old designs of equipment and hiking technique suitable for the White Mountains or the Canadian Rockies would spell disaster in the unmarked terrain of the arctic. On caribou lichen you even have to walk differently or you'll slip and fall. We put up our new tents in the yard to check them. We didn't wait until we were in the field.

In trying to achieve breakthroughs in performance, the main barrier is not people who don't try hard enough. The main barrier is the status quo design that cannot possibly do the job.

ELEMENT 5: *Insatiable curiosity and incessant search*

Now, where do these new designs come from? By definition, the status quo is the familiar; a new process must be unfamiliar. How do you get one?

By searching. The fifth key element in a system of world-class improvement is insatiable curiosity, a drive to know what you do not yet know. It starts at the top and it echoes everywhere.

When I got to Anchorage, Dr. Mandsager couldn't wait to take me on a tour of the new hospital, then still largely outlined in plasterboard and chalk markings. We spent two hours there the first time. Dick walked me through what was to become the ICU and the OR and the dental clinic. He also took me to the vast HVAC installation, explaining the problems of air exchange in a large building. He took me to the lobby and described choices of wood for the railings and tiles for the floors. He described architectural challenges in building circular spaces and open lines of sight. He spent five minutes explaining to me the design properties of the wall sconces. My point is that if you had overheard our tour, you would at various times have assumed that Dick Mandsager was an architect, a sculptor, an electrician, a heating system engineer, an interior decorator, or a security guard. You would have never, ever suspected that he was a pediatrician or, for that matter, a CEO.

This is passion. It is passionate curiosity. The status quo was to be abolished, and Dick Mandsager and his team had a passion to understand the new world they were helping to create. In fact, in some sense the senior team seemed undeniably committed to being the first people at ANMC to understand what was to come into being. I remember Sandy Haldane reporting to the senior team her recent investigations of Paul Plsek's work on creativity and how it could be applied to the move processes. I asked Dick how long he had been studying architecture and systems related to the move. "For ten years," was his answer, "maybe more."

In preparing for the Brooks Range, I visited the Anchorage office of the U.S. Geological and Geophysical Survey eight times. I became obsessed with maps and map reading. Topographical maps, of which we had twenty-six on the trip, are tough to read, especially with one-hundred-foot contour lines and no trails marked. They contain arcane symbols and lots of detailed quantitative data, but you have to know how to harvest information off the page, how to line up your compass and travel between the map and the real world. You have to understand magnetic declination and how dry stream beds in one season can be torrents in another. All of this I learned as I prepared for the Brooks Range trip. I was hungry to learn. Readings about compasses, trail foods, and bear safety replaced Stephen King and Agatha Christie at my bedside. For months before the trip, the decor of our dinner table often included a map spread out for discussion.

To invent a new world with new performance characteristics, knowledge must get into the system. There is only one door—its name is curiosity. Curiosity, beginning at the top, makes learning possible. Without it there is only control, and control is insufficient in complex system change. Gustavus Adolphus II did not understand ships. He understood power, he wanted guns, he wanted to know how the *Vasa* would look; but he did not want to know how the *Vasa* worked. He was too busy to be bothered, and his ship sank.

Separation of the intelligence of our executive leaders from the work of health care is a luxury we cannot afford. In this sense, I believe that curiosity is a nondelegable executive function. This is not intended to be rate-limiting. It is not that the CEO must know all and investigate all; that would slow us down terribly. But the executive who makes it a point to understand new systems in depth thereby models inquiry that must be a property throughout the ranks of any adaptive organization.

Let's say what we want: wait-free health care, error-free health care, scientifically based health care, the continuous reduction of waste, the continuous empowering of patients to make choices. If the ANMC move and the Brooks Range trip are to be models, then executives who seek success must begin personal inquiry into the dynamics and sciences of waits, errors, waste, and choice. They must become students of process like Richard Mandsager, who got interested in the design of wall sconces. Even more important, they must create and nurture a culture and reward system in which, to borrow the words of GE's CEO Jack Welch, "Taking an idea is better than having an idea."

ELEMENT 6: *Total relationships with customers*

One special and important form of curiosity in the service of improvement is curiosity about customers. This curiosity goes far, far beyond the classical quarterly surveys and occasional focus groups that are now traditions in health care. These will never, never get us to world class. What I have in mind is more like a continuous dance with our patients, their families, and their communities—a deep, abiding, and ceaseless effort to see the world—thoroughly—as those who depend on us see it.

For the Alaska Native Medical Center, steeped in relationship with the native population, this is not just desirable; it is their identity. Natives—the customers—don't just use the IHS; in large part they own it and, as I think it should be in all of health care, the caregivers are not the hosts but the guests of the patients. Before the senior leaders, many of them natives themselves, chose the architects of the new facility, they insisted that the candidates visit many native villages throughout Alaska. Their aim was to create a structure that would welcome people from all over the state, even those who otherwise spent their lives in villages with no buildings taller than two stories. How could the entire native community feel welcome—own—a new $160-million facility of 433,000 square feet in the outskirts of Anchorage? How could it be their place?

The answer lies in infinite attention to detail and in constant and repeated listening to native leaders at all phases of design. The entrance way is modeled on the arctic entrances of village dwellings. The clinic roofs follow the contour of native longhouses. The wall sconces are made to mimic the colors and translucence of Bering Sea ice at the time of spring breakup. Everywhere the interior spaces are circles, as are the meeting places in native cultures. Each hallway ends in windows overlooking the mountains surrounding the Anchorage bowl, so that the people inside can orient themselves, as they always do, to natural features to get their bearings. These elements of design did not come from textbooks or professional guidelines. They came, and can come, from careful listening to the people served—the co-designers of spaces and processes.

Involving customers in design is just one manifestation of a focus on total relationship with customers, or in our case, with patients, families, and communities. Bringing the patient directly into the design is one way. Simulation—experiencing the world exactly as the patient does—is another way, like my colleague Dave Gustafson did when he arranged to be admitted as a "patient" to the University of Wisconsin Hospital for "pseudo-cardiac catheterization and surgery." When it comes to getting ideas for improvement, no vantage point in health care is better than the horizontal position. I am still waiting for the first senior leadership group to take me up on my suggestion to be admitted to their own facility for three days and take notes.

Dr. Larry Staker at Latter-Day Saints (LDS) Hospital in Salt Lake City has taken the relationship with customers one step further by training his patients to make decisions on their own that normally are reserved for doctors. Dr. Staker had found that his diabetic patients were in much worse control than he had thought as he adjusted their insulin doses. He trained himself, and them, in the use of simple control charts to help them make adjustments in insulin without overadjusting, and produced much more stable patterns of blood sugar. The first figure shows anticoagulation when Dr. Staker is adjusting the Coumadin doses in one patient (Figure 6.3.A). The next figure shows the INR (international normalized ratio) in the same patient when the patient is adjusting Coumadin according to statistical process control methods (Figure 6.3.B). We've only scratched the surface of what we can do with patients once we commit to transferring knowledge and methods to them.

The bigger idea is about tacos. It is to see ourselves in relationship to the total lives of the people we serve—in all dimensions of their being and through time. At Taco Bell, I am told, the young people at the counter who give out the food are told that when a teenage customer gives them $1.39 for a taco, they are not receiving $1.39. They learn that what they are doing instead is very carefully peeling a small sticker that says "$1.39" off a large sticker attached loosely to the cus-

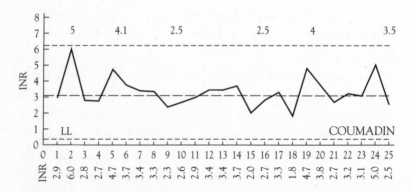

Figure 6.3.A. Anticoagulation for Atrial Fibrillation Stroke Prevention While Adjusting Coumadin Doses.
Source: Latter-Day Saints (LDS) Hospital, Salt Lake City, Utah.

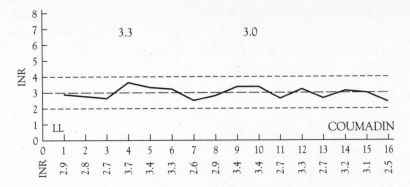

Figure 6.3.B. Anticoagulation for Atrial Fibrillation Stroke Prevention While Adjusting Coumadin According to Statistical Process Control Methods.
Source: Latter-Day Saints (LDS) Hospital, Salt Lake City, Utah.

tomer's forehead that says "$10,000," which is the amount of money that kid may spend at Taco Bell through his lifetime. Seeing our patients in terms of a disease, an admission, a visit, or even an episode of care is less sophisticated than this message from Taco Bell.[2]

ELEMENT 7: *Redefining productivity and throughput*

Which brings us to another dimension of world-class improvement—a deep understanding of what you make or, to put it more bluntly, the right definition of *throughput* or *productivity*. If in health care we make relationships, why do we count encounters and call that productivity? That would be like paying kidney specialists for their patients' urine output—it reveals a total misunderstanding of the proper definition of success.

I am not naive about the chaotic payment systems that force organizations to call visits throughput. I am just pointing out that we cannot achieve world-class improvement unless our definitions of production, and the incentives we attach to them, are aligned with the bold aims we discussed earlier. In the Brooks Range, success was only partially measured in miles per day. We also valued safety, fun, learning about plant and animal species, and great trail food. If anyone in our party had confused distance with success, he or she would have missed a great trip. King Gustavus Adolphus insisted on the number of guns the *Vasa* would carry. He counted guns. So, Gus, where's your boat now?

ELEMENT 8: *Understanding waste*

I have mentioned in past Forum speeches, and want to empha-size again, that bold aims and a commitment to dramatic improve-ment must include a deep understanding of the nature and magnitude of waste, and a commitment to drive it out. At the world-class level I see a focus on waste removal that absolutely no health care organization in my experience even begins to match. The trick is first to understand the many disguises of waste, and to develop the capacity to recognize it. A modern company sees waste in scrap materials, in motion, in inspection, in unused energy, in disorder, in inventory, in idle capital, in unused imagi-nation and ideas from the workforce, in warranty costs and repairs, in excess capacity, and in unused information. It is not uncom-mon for strong efforts over several years to recover 30 to 40 per-cent of former production costs through waste reduction. GE's overall prices have fallen 4 percent a year for ten years in a row, while in that same time its profits have risen an average of 14 per-cent per year. GE did that through globalization, market expansion, and waste reduction. In health care, I know of no organization at all that has centered its financial strategy on waste reduction, even while they complain bitterly at being held to the Consumer Price Index for their price increases.

If you want to be an expert on waste, come to the Brooks Range. For eight days, until our airdrop resupply, we had exactly what was on our backs to use—nothing more. That meant recognizing essen-tials and culling what we did not need. For example, we removed the paper labels from tea bags before we packed them. By the time

we left, I would say that our backpacks were nearly the exact opposite of the average medical record.

Here is waste. Here are the forms bins behind the secretary's
desk on the hospital ward where I teach every year (Figure 6.4).
There are seventy-eight forms here: a form for ordering a CT scan,
one for an MRI, two for pathology specimens, three for the blood
bank. There are yellowing stacks of different forms for progress notes
by physical therapists, occupational therapists, respiratory therapists, doctors, and nurses. There are two different forms here for
ordering more forms. Stacks like this—complexity like this—is long
gone from the world-class organization. They may not be hiking the
Brooks Range, but they know full well that they cannot carry this
on their backs and expect to succeed.

ELEMENT 9: *Cooperation*

All of this—including waste reduction—is at bottom about
becoming and improving a system. Systems, and bold achievements

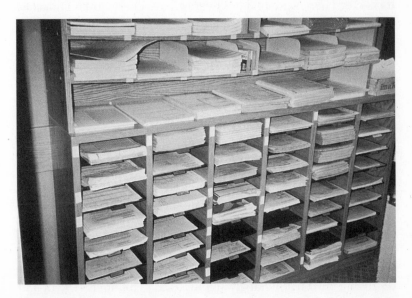

Figure 6.4. Waste (Medical Forms).

for systems, are all about interactions. And that is not yet something we are very good at. There is a sign on the door of the physicians' conference room at a hospital where I teach, and on the door of the next room there is a sign for the nurses' conference room. It's hard to find a nurse in the first, and hard to find a doctor in the second. A wall without a window separates them; it is as if they were in charge of different patients. That wall creates problems, and even more, I think it represents beliefs and traditions of separateness that are thoroughly in our way now.

Try that in the Brooks Range and you are headed for trouble. We didn't have a kids' group and a grownups' group, or a fast group and a slow group. Becca, age ten, spotted the grizzly bear first and she helped us all. We put into play rules about huddling and speaking up and staying together, because we needed them to survive. When you cross the fast-moving water of an Arctic stream, you hold onto each others' packs and form a wedge with your bodies. It keeps any one of you from being swept away.

ANMC devoted constant attention to teamness as it planned its move. There were huddles everywhere. Every other Thursday, a senior leader such as Rinna Merculieff or Frank Williams held an open meeting—an "all hands" meeting where anyone at all could come and ask questions, share ideas, and get reconnected to the whole. The senior leadership team met always in a fishbowl style, allowing anyone in the hospital to sit in and, if they wished, to comment.

The harder the goal is, the less the walls help. Thirty seamen running beam to beam on the *Vasa* almost capsized it a few days before it was launched. I guess that's something you don't tell the King because he's probably meeting in the King's conference room.

Jack Welch at GE speaks about making his company a "boundaryless organization." That's not because he is a nice guy. That's because he has breathtakingly ambitious goals for improvement and he cannot get there if the walls are too high.

ELEMENT 10: *Extreme levels of trust*

And that leads me to the last of the elements of world class that I want to mention today: trust. It is a total illusion to believe that even with the highest aims, clearest strategy, best measurements, and most capable designs, success will be in hand. Complex systems don't work that way. Great concepts still need local action—the reinvention and local embrace that I spoke about in my Forum speech last year.

In the Brooks Range, we arrived at camp each night exhausted, wet, and cold, but there was a job to do: cooking, setting up tents, scouting the area for firewood and safety hazards, planning the next day's route. No one was really in charge, but it all happened. We did it with trust. Each person or subgroup had their assignment, and we did not have the time or leisure to second-guess one another. We relied on one another.

As they did at ANMC. Move day was a ballet of individual initiative. I could say that everyone had their job to do, but it would be more correct to say that everyone *found* their job to do. At some point, inevitably, trust substituted for control, invention for instruction, free will for power, and pride for incentive. It is what Margaret Wheatley calls *self-organization*,[3] and it is inseparable from breakthrough. It's what we see here at this Forum.

The lesson about the *Vasa* is not about the risk of ambition. It is about the risk of ambition without change, ambition without method. In our lives—even in our daily lives—we do accomplish the extraordinary. You've been there: you played a great game, you reached the summit, you aced the test, you kicked the habit, you rescued someone, or you held on long enough for rescue to come. Mark Murray has done it at Kaiser, Sue Leavitt at Lawrence General, Ron Kirshner at Rochester General, and Bill Nugent at Dartmouth; and the leaders of ANMC, and Becca, Jessica, Daniel, and Benjamin Berwick in the Brooks Range, have done it. We made it because we committed, we planned, we shared, we learned, we invented, we trusted each other, and we made our own, new trail where there was none before.

Let's learn. The *Vasa* sank not because ambition is bad, but because it is not enough.

ANMC moved—without a flaw. On move day, which began at 5:30 A.M., I arrived at the old facility at 9:00 to find an empty shell. No one home. In a little more than four hours, the whole she-bang—patients, programs, staff, equipment, clinics, emergency room—everything—moved across town and was up and running. At the new place I found Dick Mandsager, CEO; Frank Williams, COO; and Mike Westley, CMO, in Dick's office sipping coffee and reminiscing about the year. The clock at Mandsager's elbow is right. It reads 10:00 on move day; 10:00 A.M. Done. Impossible. Done.

The mountains are there. Where are we? Seven drug errors per one hundred admissions? A national cesarean section rate of 24 percent? Up to almost five hundred thousand unnecessary hysterectomies a year? Patients and families waiting, pacing with unanswered questions? American medical care costs 30 percent more than care in any other system in the developed world, leaving forty million people without insurance? The wrong drugs are used to treat 25 percent of ear infections, and the right drugs are missing in the care of 80 percent of elderly victims of heart attacks?

My friends, the breeze is rising. How good is your ship?

Notes

1. Solomon, S. L., Wallace, E. M., Ford-Jones, E. L., Baker, W. M., Martone, W. J., Kopin, I. J., Critz, A. D., and Allen, J. R. "Medication Errors with Inhalant Epinephrine Mimicking an Epidemic of Neonatal Sepsis." *New England Journal of Medicine*, 1984, *310*(3), 166–170.

2. Applegate, L. M., Schlesinger, L. A., and Delong, D. "Taco Bell, Inc., 1983–94." Harvard Business School case, May 2, 1998.

3. Wheatley, M. J. *Leadership and the New Science: Learning About Organization from an Orderly Universe.* San Francisco: Berrett-Koehler, 1992.

7

Eagles and Weasels

Commentary

Paul Plsek

Do you know what it's like to climb Mount Everest?

In 1998, the same year that Donald Berwick gave the tenth anniversary National Forum speech that you are about to read, author Jon Krakauer made that climb and documented the journey in his best-selling nonfiction novel, *Into Thin Air*.

Krakauer described what it was like to ascend almost twenty thousand feet, only to realize that he had an additional ten thousand feet and the most challenging part of the climb still to go. Among the difficulties he encountered were fear bordering on panic, a sense of dizziness, terrible headaches, loss of appetite, exhaustion, and mental dullness.

Come to think of it, if you were a health care leader interested in improvement in 1998, you probably *did* know what it was like to climb Mount Everest.

Prior to Edmund Hillary and Tenzing Norgay's ascent in 1953, reaching the top of Mount Everest was an impossible dream. After their ascent, the world realized that we only *thought* it was impossible because no one had yet done it. Since then, hundreds have repeated the feat. Authors such as Krakauer remind us of pioneers like Hillary and Norgay and tell us the stories of the many who followed, precisely to remind us that seemingly impossible achievements are possible.

It was in that great storytelling tradition that Berwick riveted the audience at the Institute for Healthcare Improvement's 10th Annual National Forum with his "Eagles and Weasels" speech. Berwick acknowledged to us on that day that the first decade of concerted effort to improve health care had been hard work, but he also pointed out that even more challenges lie ahead. It would have been easy to suggest it was time to rest on the many accomplishments of that day. Many would have commented that we would do well to be more realistic, that we should face the fact that while truly transforming the whole health care delivery system was an important dream, it was just a bit far-fetched given our experiences to that point. Like Krakauer's recounting of climbs up Everest, Berwick's retelling of the battle against leukemia drove home the point that what we might have thought was impossible—winning a seemingly hopeless battle in the improvement of care—had in fact been done before, and hence could be done again.

It was just the message that all of us in the health care improvement movement needed to hear that day.

Not only was Berwick inspirational as he addressed his audience in 1998, he was also once again practicing time travel. Defying the laws of physics, Berwick always seems to know already the topics we will all be talking about several years later. In this speech, for example, you will find ideas about social movements, whole-systems thinking, broadscale spread of improvement ideas, communities of practice, knowledge management, and social justice. You could not attend workshops on those topics at the 1998 National Forum because practically no one—except Berwick—was talking about them then. Four years later you can explore the leading edge of these topics at the 2002 National Forum because lots of people are talking about them now.

Improving health care and climbing Mount Everest have a lot in common. It has been hard work to get this far and will perhaps be even harder work to go further. But with visionary leaders like Berwick guiding the improvement movement, I think we will be just fine. On that day in December 1998, we were all reenergized to adjust our packs, relace our boots, and continue the climb.

Eagles and Weasels

10th Annual National Forum on Quality Improvement in Health Care

Orlando, Florida, December 6, 1998

The first National Forum of the Institute for Healthcare Improvement (IHI), held in Boston, Massachusetts, in June 1989, attracted just under three hundred people—hardy souls—a fringe element in health care interested in the premise that there might be systematic approaches to improving care that we could study, learn, and apply for the benefit of our patients and society. At this, the tenth Forum, we are nearly three thousand strong and represent what has become a vast and promising movement in health care, nearly worldwide, with the same premise but much more sophistication and experience than we could possibly have imagined in 1989—only ten years ago.

We should celebrate our work. You here, and the hundreds of organizations and thousands of people with whom you share this improvement work, are, I firmly believe, the best resource and the greatest hope for positive change that our health care system has to draw upon. We have not yet come fully into our own—there is much more work to do—but when we take the perspective of a decade, it becomes remarkably easy to see how amazing our progress together has been.

I'd like to reflect a bit on where we've been, and on where we have yet to travel. Recently in the same week I received two quotes on my desk that, taken together, summarize a lot about how I view the IHI and our work together. The first quote came from

Keynote speech presented at the 10th Annual National Forum on Quality Improvement in Health Care, Orlando, Florida, December 6, 1998.

Joanne Lynn. Joanne is probably the leading advocate in the nation for the improvement of care at the end of life. She chaired the IHI's Breakthrough Series Collaborative on that topic, and frankly she is one of my heroes. Joanne sent me a bookmark on which was printed these words: "Sometimes you just have to jump off the cliff and build your wings on the way down."[1] That's exactly how it felt to be at the table in the late 1980s with the founding group of the IHI. We proposed a psychotic mission: to improve health care in the United States and Canada—period. As if to confirm our psychosis, two years ago we removed the North American restriction and embraced what I firmly hope and believe will become a global objective: better care on the planet. Other planets will follow.

A few days later, on my birthday, my son Ben sent me an e-mail with some other quotes, one of which read, "Eagles may soar, but weasels don't get sucked into jet engines."

It's a choice. Eagle: jump and grow your wings. Or weasel: hunker down and stay safe. We chose eagle.

Was it wise? We don't know yet. We've made a good start. Improvements—a lot of improvements—are now visible. But our wings are stubby and the job undone seems overwhelming. We formed the IHI to close gaps, and the gaps remain. And they are very, very big gaps.

As when the IHI began, it is still true today that many American patients receive care they do not need, while others never get the care that could help them. Our national cesarean section rate remains well above 20 percent—as high as 40 percent in some areas—despite America's scientifically supported, professionally espoused goal of 10 percent or less. More than 30 percent of children with simple ear infections receive powerful and toxic antibiotics that they do not need. We do more than six hundred thousand hysterectomies each year in our nation—as many as 80 percent of which are unnecessary—and even more unnecessary coronary angioplasties. Six out of every one hundred patients in American hospitals are harmed or nearly harmed by a medication error sometime during their admission. More than half of the elderly people who could benefit from pneumococcal immunization fail to get it, and even though bicycle helmets could cut head injuries in children by 80 percent, only 12 percent of American kids wear bicycle helmets. Teenage smoking rates have risen in the past ten years by almost 50 percent. American patients have developed tough skin for long waiting times for appointments and in doctors' offices, for increasing bureaucratic barriers to specialty care, and for confusion as they migrate among the sites and caregivers in our complex technical care system. American doctors and nurses bear an increasing burden of precertification rituals, forms, and administrative review as they guide their patients through care—many doctors tell me they now spend as much as 20 or 25 percent of their time in such review and authorization processes, even while the demands on them for productivity and throughput rise.

And the biggest quality problem of all in our nation is still there: injustice—inequity. We have at least forty million uninsured Americans, and as many underinsured. The biggest risk factors for early death and poor health in our nation today are ethnicity and poverty.

These problems are immense. Pollyannas of improvement can relabel them "opportunities," but that's a bit of a trick. This list of needed improvements seems relentless, discouraging, and all too familiar. It is easy to lose heart.

And it is getting even easier to lose heart. Even as we have learned to make improvements step by step, the bigger victories—the ones we really need—seem out of our reach. In the IHI's Breakthrough Series, we have now learned how to help teams from organizations reliably make project-by-project improvements. We can tackle a problem such as medication errors, waiting times, unnecessary drug use, or better asthma care, and help make significant local gains in about two out of every three organizations that participate. The local gains are big: a clinic reduces its waiting times by 80 percent; a hospital reduces its unnecessary use of albumen by 95 percent; a nursing unit cuts medication errors in half. This is good stuff.

But it is not enough. Not nearly enough. The system as a whole remains stuck. We have not yet found a way to scale improvement up to the system level, to spread sound changes into all the corners of our work, and to place improvement where it belongs: at the core. The theme of the 1998 Forum, "Power of Ten," is all about the issue of scale. It is not about where we have been; it is about where we must go.

But ambitious aims scare us away. As health care reels into the twenty-first century, it seems naive to pursue fundamental improvements of performance. Just getting through the day seems accomplishment enough. System after system continues to face tens of millions of dollars of operating losses; more and more plans consider dropping Medicaid and Medicare contracts; doctors fight for time and control. Where can we possibly find the energy to power up improvements when the energy drain is so great? Really and truly, can we succeed in shaping health care as we need it to become?

At times like this it's the weasels who seem smart. But they're not so smart. Weasels lack perspective. They're too close to the ground. It keeps them away from jet engines, but all they can see is holes. Can't we find a better image? What makes eagles, anyway?

My mentor, Tom Nolan, has, as is often the case, supplied a framework for thinking about big tasks, big shifts—hope. It's a simple framework, but very powerful. Tom says that a big shift—the sort of social change and new accomplishments that health care needs—requires assets of three types. He calls these *will*, *ideas*, and *execution*. His model parallels the pathfinding work of Dave Gustafson, another mentor of mine, on leadership of change, which Gustafson says requires "tension for change" (or will), a "plausible, superior alternative to the status quo" (or ideas), and "self-efficacy skills, resources, and social supports" (or elements of execution). Whenever Gustafson and Nolan agree with each other, I tend to say, "Yes, sir—of course, sir." Let's take their model seriously and parse our future work.

But first I want to look back with you not ten years or twenty, but nearly thirty years, to 1968. That year, fresh from college, I became a medical student, and to help support myself I got a job as the night technician in the blood bank of the Children's Hospital in Boston, where I would later train. In the dark hours of the early morning, a phone would ring and a transport worker would appear in the blood bank with a vial of blood, often from a young child on Division 28, the leukemia ward. I still recall their names—Bobby, Alan, Jeff—and I still recall the image of their blood smears in my microscope—torn, malignant blast cells of acute lymphoblastic leukemia, blood deficient in vital elements such as platelets—the blood of dying children.

My job was to cross-match replacement blood or platelet supplements, but it was nearly futile work. Almost all of these children would die. It was only a matter of time. I was twenty-three years old, and I remember trying to understand emotionally what I was dealing with—as if at twenty-three I ever could. I got into the habit of carrying the cross-matched blood myself up to the ward so I could see the children whose names I had typed on the labels, giving them faces and talking sometimes with a few of them. And one by one, as the weeks and months passed, their names would disappear from the order sheets.

In the 1938 edition of Porter and Carter's textbook, *Management of the Sick Infant and Child,* the three-page chapter on leukemia states, "Death in acute leukemia is a matter of days or weeks. . . . No form of treatment is of the slightest use. . . . Repeated transfusions are sometimes employed, but they only serve to prolong a miserable existence for a little while."[2]

It was pretty much the same in the fourth edition of Nelson's *Textbook of Pediatrics,* published the year I was born, 1946: "Because the disease is invariably fatal, treatment should be directed toward modifying the symptoms so that the patient may enjoy relative comfort."[3]

By 1954, in the sixth edition of Nelson's *Textbook,* the first glimmers of work on chemotherapy began to show. "Leukemia is a universally fatal disease," it starts, but then it mentions the new folic acid antagonists and says, "With the administration of these antimetabolites, from 25 percent to 50 percent of children with acute leukemia experience complete remissions." But the remissions were always temporary: "Ultimately leukemia becomes unresponsive to any currently available agent."

And the seventh edition, in 1959, says, "With supportive antileukemic therapy, life can be prolonged in the majority of instances for months to a year or so."

Sixteen years later, 1975, in the tenth edition of Nelson's *Textbook*, look what we find: "Substantial numbers of children with acute lymphoblastic leukemia are alive and in remission more than three years after initial diagnosis. There is mounting optimism that some of these patients may never relapse and thus represent cure." Mounting optimism.

By 1986 you could pick up Nelson's twelfth edition and read this: "There is now sufficient evidence with patients having common ALL—Acute Lymphocytic Leukemia—who have achieved longterm disease-free intervals after cessation of therapy to indicate that with current regimens a patient who has been in complete remission for six years or more has a very small likelihood of later relapse."

1986 is actually a very important year for me. That year Blan Godfrey and I first met, got our grant from the John A. Hartford Foundation, and convened the National Demonstration Project on Quality Improvement in Health Care. That year we planted the seeds that would become the IHI—although we didn't know it at the time.

But 1986 is also an important year for another, more private reason. It's the year I met Joshua. He was fifteen years old and he was not on my schedule. He was an emergency. The nurse practitioner I worked with, Jan, pulled me into exam room three. "You better take a look at this kid—he's hurting."

He *was* hurting. Joshua was lying on his back on the exam table writhing in pain—back pain—and screaming obscenities I had never heard before. Young adolescents usually don't have bad back pain and I couldn't figure out what was going on. In my haste I missed his enormously enlarged spleen, and only that night, when our laboratory finally woke me up at home, did I finally get the diagnosis right. His blood smear was full of blast cells. Joshua had acute lymphoblastic leukemia, and his back pain was from the cancer invading the marrow spaces in the bones of his spine. I had the wrong diagnosis. He hadn't wrenched his back; he was dying.

So, the next morning I was sitting in the hospital with Joshua and his mother, explaining what was ahead. The story I told, and the saga that followed, are too long to fit into this speech. Basically, Joshua got world-class initial treatment for his leukemia, exactly at what we would call today the "best practice" standard, and predictably he went into remission. But he relapsed. In, say, 1968, when I was in the blood bank, relapse was a certain death sentence. But not in 1986.

When Joshua relapsed, the American medical care system went into full gear. Within weeks of his relapse he was in remission again, and I had him scheduled for a bone marrow transplant in one of the finest centers in the world. Two months later he was transplanted with his brother's marrow at the "best practice" standard of care. There were complications, but Joshua survived. A posttransplant course is never simple; it requires a lot of cooperation, surveillance, and prompt responses to complications. But he made it.

In fact, I spoke with Joshua yesterday to check this speech out with him. He says "Hi." He's twenty-eight years old. No signs of leukemia.

When I worked in the Children's Hospital blood bank, almost all children with acute lymphoblastic leukemia died. Today, almost all live. We built wings.

How?

Don't expect a neat and simple story of how; there isn't one. At one level it's too complicated to explain. Here are some elements.

First, there is *science*. In the building next to the Children's Hospital blood bank I worked in, long before I ever got there, the lights had been burning for two decades in the laboratories of Dr. Sidney Farber. Dr. Farber believed in the possibility of selective poisoning of the cancer cells of leukemia, and he worked out the metabolic pathways he learned to interrupt with drugs, initially aminopterin, then methotrexate, then others. Trial after trial, patient by patient, Dr. Farber and his colleagues discovered the exact, tightrope doses of chemotherapeutic agents that were just enough to kill most of the leukemia cells while not harming normal cells too much.

Of course his work would not have been possible without a long and simultaneous network of science worldwide developing better understanding of the folic acid metabolism pathways that Dr. Farber wanted to attack, or developing and offering options among possible selective chemotherapeutic agents to try. Their work was published, exchanged, discussed at meetings, criticized—and knowledge grew.

In 1955, Dr. C. Gordon Zubrod brought a team of young clinical scientists to the National Cancer Institute (NCI) at the National Institutes of Health (NIH) to develop cures for cancer. They built on Dr. Farber's work. I talked the week before last with the man who headed that team in 1955, Dr. Tom Frei. At age thirty-five, Dr. Frei became the chief of medicine at NCI and organized himself and his colleagues for an all-out assault on leukemia. In 1955, when they started, it was neither easy nor obvious that they'd win. Remember what that 1954 textbook said: "Leukemia is a universally fatal disease. . . ."

Dr. Frei said to me, "We went into this with the thought that we would try to cure the disease over time"; but he also told me that most of his close colleagues from throughout the world were telling him that the goal was hopeless, that he was throwing his career away on an impossible aim. All children with leukemia died.

Step by step, Dr. Frei and his team wore away at the fatal statistics. They learned first how to induce remissions more and more reliably, then how to lengthen those remissions by combinations of drugs and by treatment *during* remission. They learned how to support the children with platelet transfusions and proper management of infections while their bone marrow was depressed by treatment, and they learned to attack residual cancer cells in the spinal fluid—which was what they called "a pharmacological sanctuary," where cancer cells could not be reached by intravenous drugs.

At first only the remission rates changed: 20 percent in 1955, 40 percent in 1959, 90 percent by the early 1960s. But the remissions were temporary; almost all patients still died, albeit after longer and longer disease-free intervals. As of the early 1960s, at most 5 to 10 percent seemed to be truly cured, and nobody was sure that those few survivals had anything to do with treatment.

But as central nervous system treatment became more and more aggressive, the apparent cure rate finally began to rise. It crept up over 20 percent by the late 1960s, and rose steadily after that. With ongoing refinements of dosages, routes, and supportive management, today more than 75 percent of childhood ALL is cured, and for some subtypes the cure rate is well over 90 percent.

Of course none of that scientific progress would have mattered had there not been a tightly linked national community of caregivers—hematologists, pediatricians, and others—who knew that leukemia was an enemy and who were willing to become part of the search for a cure by referring patients to clinical trials, pooling data on outcomes, and studying together so that the cycle times from NCI's laboratory to applications in the field were minimized.

The research was coordinated on a national basis, involving not just NCI but also Roswell Park, Harvard, St. Jude's, and many other clinical laboratories. It was a national learning system with a hub at NCI. Even today, 80 to 90 percent of all children with ALL participate in clinical trials, as do 60 percent of all children with cancer. (That's compared, by the way, to 2 to 3 percent of all adults with cancer. As Joseph Simone and Jane Lyons wrote recently, "These percentages mean that 6 or 7 of every 10 children with cancer contribute in a systematic way to improving care, while such information from 19 of 20 adults with cancer is simply lost.")[4]

This could not have been done if there hadn't been payers committed to seeing progress made. Not just philanthropists, but day-to-day health care payers and insurers who understood that the boundary between "standard care" and the growth of knowledge is artificial, moving, and a function only of our ignorance. Leukemia researchers and caregivers got paid to help improve. Learning was part of the work.

None of that would have mattered if the general community of caregivers and organizations had been satisfied with the then-current performance levels. You see, leukemia *was* fatal, but some people—actually, only a few people—thought that surrender to that fact was not an option. Dr. Frei and his colleagues were simply not willing to give up. They insisted on reading the doom pronounced in the 1954 sixth edition of Nelson's *Textbook*—"universally fatal"—as a description only of *current* possibilities, but not as a limit on *future* ones. They refused to explain to all future victims of leukemia that expecting to live was unrealistic. They fought disease, not expectations.

I cannot characterize my feelings at 3 A.M. in the darkness of the blood bank in 1968 as anything but hopeless. I was twenty-three years old. I sometimes could not read the slides through my tears. I felt hopeless, but just enough people were not hopeless. On the contrary, a movement was afoot—reflected in the cooperative, dedicated, consistent, and sometimes selfless endeavors of coordinated people and institutions, some of whom never met each other at all, but all of whom shared an aim and would not let it go. The work was not bounded. It took place *in* organizations, but the actual work system was *among* organizations. Organizations were not ends; they were means. The purpose ruled.

In Tom Nolan's terms, there was *will*. Not will everywhere, but enough of it to sustain the work. Just enough people. Just enough will. There was strong, insistent leadership—constancy of purpose—in Gordon Zubrod and others. They convened a close-knit team that knew the job. They developed clear results measurement, first by defining remission formally and figuring out how to diagnose it with bone marrow tests. Their psychology was, in Dr. Zubrod's words, "Every success uncovers the next obstacle." Obstacles were not stopping points; they were direction finders. And they held a long-term view of the aim. The NCI team proposed using platelet transfusions in 1957 because kids in remission were dying of bleeding, but the head of the NIH Blood Bank refused to supply the platelets. "Remember why we're here," Tom Frei remembers him saying. "We're going to cure leukemia. Every success uncovers the next obstacle. Bleeding is simply the next obstacle." Then he said he would start his own damn blood bank at NCI if NIH's wouldn't work with him. He got the platelets, and of the first fifteen children who got them, 92 percent stopped bleeding, compared with 9 percent of untreated patients. That's will.

Then there are *ideas*. In the laboratories of NCI and extending to many other research institutions and into protocol networks throughout the country, the ideas were developing. These willful change agents worked with strong theories, and then they refined those ideas with progressive, cumulative tests.

The ideas did not belong to anyone. They were a good in common. All through this time the investigators linked their knowledge across many sites, and they continually scanned for ideas in related but foreign domains. An arthritis researcher in Texas noticed that hydrocortisone in arthritis patients reduced their lymphocyte counts. Within a couple of weeks Dr. Frei not only knew about that observation, but he was beginning to test steroids as adjuncts in the treatment of lymphocytic leukemia. He didn't say, "Arthritis is different." He said, "There is similarity here and maybe I can use it to help my patients."

You can see the progress of ideas in this graph, from a wonderful book by John Laszlo (Figure 7.1). These are survival curves for children with ALL in successive waves of research protocols through three decades. At first, all die. Then slowly, protocol after protocol, the curves decelerate, and then flatten. In the 1996 fifteenth edition of Nelson's *Textbook*, after reporting the cure rate of over 70 percent, you find these words: "treatment is the single most important prognostic factor." Remember the fourth edition, in 1946? "Because the disease is invariably fatal, treatment should

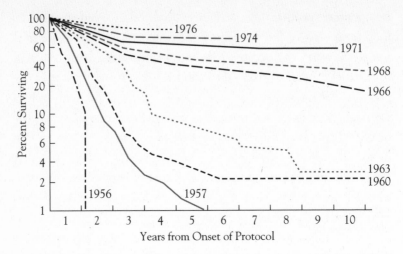

Figure 7.1. Acute Lymphocytic Leukemia Survival in Children under Twenty.

Source: Laszlo, J., *The Cure of Childhood Leukemia: Into the Age of Miracles* (New Brunswick, N.J.: Rutgers University Press, 1995, p. 228). Used by permission of Rutgers University Press.

be directed toward modifying the symptoms so that the patient may enjoy relative comfort." Now treatment is the single most important prognostic factor.

The next figure illustrates the progress of ideas in tabular form (Figure 7.2). In 1955, single drug chemotherapy achieved a 20 percent remission rate. In 1957, multiple drugs were achieving 45 percent remissions. Platelet transfusions in 1957 stopped 92 percent of the bleeding. By 1959, treatment in remission was achieving ten-month remissions, and drug dose increases got it to fifteen months. The first apparent cures appeared with four-drug treatment in 1962 (15 percent cures), and central nervous system relapses fell from 60 percent to 20 percent of patients when drugs were used in the spinal fluid. By 1968, St. Jude's was using brain irradiation and reporting a 35 percent cure rate, which rose steadily as dosages and supports were fine-tuned, all the way to 80 percent cure for some forms of ALL by 1995.

1955	Chemotherapy	20% remission
1957	Multiple drugs	45% remission
1957	Platelet support	92% stop bleeding
1959	Rx in remission	10-month remission
1961	Full-dose drugs	15-month remission
1962	VAMP regimen	10%–15% cure
1963	CNS drugs	CNS relapse 60%–20%
1968	CNS X-ray	35% cure
1995	Multiagent Rx	75%–80% cure

Figure 7.2. The Progress of Ideas.

Source: Laszlo, J., *The Cure of Childhood Leukemia: Into the Age of Miracles*. (New Brunswick, N.J.: Rutgers University Press, 1995.) Used by permission of Rutgers University Press.

So first there is will. Then there are ideas. But none of these would really have mattered to Joshua without *execution*. All of the ideas in the world couldn't help if people did not accept—universally accept—change. Leukemia was treated one way—unsuccessfully—in 1955, a different way—slightly more successfully—in 1965, and a new way again in 1975, and so on. Every single time, the care system had to change to keep up with the knowledge. The rising rates of success were not bottled up in laboratories. This was not a change that stopped with prototypes. It *spread*. Throughout the story—at least by the mid-1960s—the best practices in leukemia care were not rare; they were the national standard.

The will and ideas would not have mattered at all to Joshua if that universal deployment of change had not been part of the picture. The virtual defeat of ALL did not stop at the laboratory door or the walls of St. Jude's. Throughout the war, the army fighting against leukemia developed and then refined nationwide networks of referral, learning, and communication. By the time I was searching for an available bone marrow transplant bed for Joshua, he and I had totally acceptable options in Seattle, Boston, and Baltimore; and though there were minor differences in approach, they all shared a central, consistent standard of care and practice—state of the art—that linked them in a common frame of shared knowledge. This was the opposite of a tower of Babel, and it is, on the whole, very nearly the opposite of the pace of spread of system improvements in health care today. The best was the standard, payers paid for improvements, there was a strong intellectual hub at NCI, and in essence the entire system of work—the nation as a whole— became a unified laboratory for continual learning.

To a remarkable degree—in fact, I find it thrilling—the treatment system for ALL in the United States today is a single system. New York or Boston, Omaha or Traverse City, urban or rural, small center or large—you can count on it. Cure: brought to *you*, Joshua, by will, ideas, and execution.

Joshua was cured. His care has cost well over $300,000. He got intensive treatment for three years, and ten more years of follow-up. He has seen easily one hundred doctors, in three major medical centers, an HMO, and several community health centers, and he has had more than a dozen hospitalizations. His medical record in only one of the hospitals has five volumes, which stack thirty inches tall and weigh collectively eighteen pounds. In one admission alone, just after his transplant, I counted 2,400 laboratory tests. But he is cured.

In 1955 Joshua would have lived for six weeks after his diagnosis. In 1960 he would have lived six months. In 1965, eighteen months, with a 15 percent chance of cure. In 1975 he had a 50 percent chance of cure. In 1985 his chances were over 70 percent. Success.

But now let me tell you the rest of Joshua's story—which I do with his permission.

Joshua is black. He was born and raised in one of the poorest areas of Boston. His home at age fifteen, when I first met him, lay just out of sight from the top floor of the medical center where he got his bone marrow transplant, but it could just as well have been on a different continent for all those two places bore in common.

I remember making a house call in 1987 to discuss his transplant options with him and his mother. His home was the only building standing in an otherwise vacant, weed-choked lot in Dorchester. I walked past a line of hookers and drug dealers not fifty yards from his front door, as he did every day of his young life. By age twelve Joshua owned his first handgun. By age fourteen he had committed his first felony. He started on cocaine at thirteen and was selling it two years later. For a while, unknown to me, during the darkest times after his bone marrow transplant, he hoarded Percocet, a narcotic, and became addicted to it for two years.

Joshua has been in the hospital eight times in the ten years since his transplant—three times for complications of his transplant, and five times for treatment of cocaine and heroin addiction. He has been arrested twice, and in 1987, the year after he was diagnosed with leukemia, he saw his oldest brother murdered by a shotgun blast through the front door of his mother's apartment.

We speak often, Joshua and I. Across a chasm we are friends, I guess. But he is frightened, and so am I. What afflicts him is bigger than both of us. And it seems relentless, overwhelmingly powerful, inevitable in its consequences, like leukemia—not leukemia *now*, but leukemia *then*—when I worked in the blood bank. "I know I am going to die," he tells me. He means die young. And he is not talking about cancer.

This year, from the Harvard Center on the Global Burden of Disease has come a report authored by Chris Murray on inequities in health.[5] Worldwide, the variation in life expectancy among nations is thirty-nine years—from an average age at death of 81 in Japan to an average age of forty-two in Sierra Leone. Within the United States, the range for men is from seventy-eight years in parts of Utah and Colorado to sixty-one years in Native American counties in rural South Dakota—a seventeen-year difference in longevity. A boy of Joshua's ethnicity born today in our nation has a life expectancy eight years shorter than that of a white child. Think about it. I don't know this for sure but my reading of the data suggests to me that getting some subtypes of acute lymphoblastic leukemia today may not shorten a child's life expectancy as much as being born black does. A black male born today in Washington, D.C., St. Louis, or New York has a life expectancy of fifty-nine years or less.

There is more. As much as Joshua's story of cancer survival is testimony to the brilliant potential we have to solve tough, tough problems, it testifies equally to other chronic, unsolved, daunting systemic problems that we have not yet mustered the will, ideas, and execution to cure. He is walking evidence both of what we *can* do and of what we *must* do.

In 1989, two years after Joshua's bone marrow transplant, his father died of a heart attack from untreated hypertension. Almost one-third of the hypertension in America today is inadequately treated.

In 1994, three years after we started the IHI, I stood with Joshua at the graveside of his mother, who died of multiple myeloma—diagnosed too late and treated inadequately at first. Her final weeks of illness were a nightmare as she was subjected to intensive care, with her pain poorly controlled, and put through invasive, painful, and undignified interventions that she had asked not to get. She had totally futile bowel surgery only a few weeks before she died. Joanne Lynn will tell you that end-of-life care in the United States is far, far from what it could be. Hundreds of thousands of patients die in pain that they do not need to suffer, and millions have futile, unwanted, and costly treatments in stages of illness where those treatments make no sense at all.

You may find this hard to believe but Joshua almost died only once during his entire twelve years of treatment, and it was not from either leukemia or chemotherapy. His heart stopped and he had to be resuscitated one night in the hospital where he had received his chemotherapy a year earlier, because he received a dose of a drug, Bactrim, that he was known to be severely allergic to and that he got anyway, again, causing anaphylaxis. We saved him, and then we almost killed him. Lucian Leape (a health policy analyst whose research has focused on error prevention and appropriateness of care) will tell you how prevalent drug errors are and how clear are the ideas we now have about how to reduce them, if only we had the will and the systems to spread effective changes.

These are cancers, too—ethnic inequities in health status, missed opportunities for prevention, unnecessary treatments given, pain not controlled, and pervasive, avoidable errors in our daily work. But you cannot show these cancers on the slide of a blood smear. The enemy has no photograph. I have no slide to show the meaning of a hundred thousand deaths each year in American hospitals due to avoidable errors such as the one that almost killed Joshua. I cannot show a photograph of what it means that more than 70 percent of dying Americans suffer inadequate pain control in the last days of their illness; or of the wages of indignity and confusion among patients whose questions go unanswered in our hospitals; or of the missed opportunities to provide effective, simple preventive and curative care to heart attack victims not given aspirin and beta blockers, elderly people not given pneumococcal vaccine, smokers not counseled by their doctors to stop smoking; or of the waste and toxicity of advanced antibiotics used where they can do no good at all, or hysterectomies performed without hope of benefit to patients. These gaps in performance are real. They harm people. They are fully documented in our health services research literature.

There is good news. If the formula for change is will, ideas, and execution, then let us notice the abundance, not just the shortages. Our strongest suit is ideas. In the work of the IHI we would have a hard time tackling almost any of these serious, unsolved problems without quickly discovering gems among us—local, proven changes; published journal papers documenting exciting alternative approaches; teachers and experts frustrated not by what they do not know but by their inability to get anyone to listen to them. I recommend, again, the work of Lucian Leape, and of the National Patient Safety Foundation at the American Medical Association. There you will find—open, for free, on their Web site—ideas for reducing medication errors that are nearly guaranteed to work. If you want to improve end-of-life care and think that ideas are lacking, spend five minutes with Joanne Lynn and you will find an agenda ready for use.

Do we lack will? Maybe. I see no national consensus now that the intolerable, embarrassing ethnic gap in morbidity and mortality must be closed. It must be closed. We are nearly alone among developed nations in our failure to commit to health care as a human right. Our will does look a little shabby.

But I am much more optimistic than that. After all, you are here. We are twenty-six hundred who intend to make change. And Tom Frei started with, maybe, twenty. Our system is in chaos, and that may be the best time of all for the few who really want their effect to multiply.

Execution is the toughest of all. We lack connections. Within a matter of days Tom Frei was using knowledge about treating arthritis in Texas to help cure kids with leukemia in Maryland. Joshua did not have to go to Memphis to get the benefit of St. Jude's protocol for brain irradiation; he got it in Boston.

Our connections are frayed by fear, by senseless competition against one another, by fragmented payment systems, and by fossilized traditions of professional isolation. We would rather reinvent something ourselves than learn what someone else knows. And we are far quicker to point out differences than to search for similarities.

We can end all of that here. Right now, if you choose. The IHI's vision statement is "to be a premier integrative force for improvement." We exist so that you can meet on common ground, with common aims, finding common will, treating ideas as a common good, and fighting in your own way the common battle against defects in our work with the same passion, intensity, and wisdom with which Tom Frei and his lunatic band of eagles at NCI fought and won the impossible battle against a hopeless disease.

You must reject the forces of nonsense. Let's choose Tom Frei and Gordon Zubrod as our models—not those who continue to insist that expecting better outcomes, more dignity in care, less waste, more safety, and more listening are unrealistic aims. You must not give in to the present. You must not agree that promises are foolish and that progress is too costly. You must not agree with those who claim that we must fight against one another to make progress for all. You must not agree that the world is too complex to improve, or that those we serve must get used to our defects. You must find the will, uncover the ideas, and absolutely insist that the best become the standard everywhere.

It would be easier to give up. I know. I told you, weasels don't get sucked into jet engines. The gaps we have yet to close seem so vast and tentacular. What afflicts our systems of care—the barriers to cure—seem so far from our reach. What is killing Joshua today seems so big. It all makes curing leukemia look like duck soup.

But trust me: if you had joined me in the blood bank in 1968, looking down on the cancer cells of doomed children, you would have felt discouraged and hopeless too, and you would have been wrong.

It can be the same with these cancers. No one called the war on leukemia "quality improvement," but it was. No one said that those who beat it were "systems thinkers," but they were. No one said then—at least not often—that they worked with shared vision, were strategically aligned, self-organizing, committed to quality, learning from variation, using guidelines, inspired by leaders, sophisticated about incentives, building on pride and joy, or customer focused. But they were. Improvement works. Systematic, collective, mission-driven, scientifically guided, evidence-based, leadership-activated, participative change works.

I know that it is hard. But if we don't try, who will? I remain convinced that somewhere deep in the heart of this nearly derailed, perilously wandering health care industry lies the reservoir of will and energy we need to cure the ills that afflict Joshua's life, not just his blood. I remain convinced that under a crust of nonsensical, aimless, enervating restructuring, accusation, surveillance, and blame, this health care community still can find in itself the intense commitment to service that cured leukemia and can likewise cure the defects that afflict our *systems* of care and that prevent us from widespread continual reduction of the total burden of illness.

Let us be very careful, very humble, before we have the audacity to declare any of these afflictions "incurable." That's for weasels. The IHI was brought into being as an organization based on the firm conviction that what is unhealed today may be healed tomorrow. We say, "Take the leap. We'll build our wings on the way down."

Leap. Leap. No weasels here. We'll build our wings on the way down.

Notes

1. Paraphrase of Ray Bradbury: "Go to the edge of the cliff and jump off. Build your wings on the way down." *Brown Daily Herald*. March 24, 1995.

2. Porter, L., and Carter, W. E. *Management of the Sick Infant and Child*. St. Louis: Mosby, 1938, 338.

3. Nelson, W. E. *Textbook of Pediatrics*. Philadelphia: Saunders, 1946, 904.

4. Simone, J. V., and Lyons, J. "Superior Cancer Survival in Children Compared to Adults: A Superior System of Cancer Care?" Background paper. Washington, D.C.: Institute of Medicine of the National Academies, 1998.

5. Murray, C.J.L., and Lopez, A. (eds.). *The Global Burden of Disease: A Comprehensive Assessment of Mortality and Disability from Diseases, Injuries, and Risk Factors in 1990 and Projected to 2020*. World Health Organization and World Bank Global Burden of Disease and Injury Series, Vol. 1. Cambridge, Mass.: Harvard University Press, 1996.

8

Escape Fire

Commentary

Karl E. Weick

What keeps people from jumping into Donald Berwick's escape fire? Why do people hold on to their heavy tools, lose agility, and endanger coworkers and patients? Those same wildland firefighters who gave Berwick some of his more compelling images also provide some answers about why the escape fire remains empty.

Since 1990, twenty-three firefighters in four separate incidents, refused to drop their tools when ordered to do so, were overrun by fire, and died with their tools beside them.[1] They died within sight of safety zones that could have been reached if they had been lighter and moved faster. For example, at the South Canyon disaster outside Glenwood Springs, Colorado, fourteen firefighters were killed on July 6, 1994, when they failed to outrun a fire that exploded through a flammable stand of Gambel oak just below them. One firefighter, whose body was found a mere 250 feet from safety at the top of the ridge, was still wearing a backpack and still had a chain saw handle in his hand, with the chain saw immediately above his right hand.

Why didn't he drop his tools? Why don't Berwick's colleagues drop theirs? Careful analysis of firefighter interviews, witness depositions, field observation, accident investigations, and computer simulations suggests answers. Some of the answers are obvious. These can be illustrated using the South Canyon fire as an example. First, the exploding fire was so loud that the crew may not have heard the order to drop their tools. Second, they were strung out in single file, and because the fire was behind them and they did not turn around, when they were told to drop their tools there was no obvious reason that they should do so. Third, because the people who ordered the firefighters to drop their tools were not familiar, the retreating crew had no reason to trust the order even if they heard it.[2] Fourth, because people sometimes survive fires by using a fire shelter, and because these shelters are safest when deployed in an area that is cleared of underbrush, they may have kept their tools to clear a safe area. Fifth, the firefighters were tired, hungry, dehydrated, and had ingested considerable carbon monoxide, all of which made it more difficult for them to think clearly, no matter what they heard. And sixth, the firefighters had little experience converting a reduction in the weight of their equipment into a gain in speed. Post hoc calculations suggest that if the people at South Canyon had covered six to nine more inches per second when they started to retreat, they would have made it to safety. But people in the crew had no way of knowing this. And when you face escalating events, it surely must feel unlikely that changes this small can make a big enough difference to matter. Thus people may refuse to drop their tools and jump into an escape fire because of deficiencies in hearing, rationale, trust, control, physical well-being, and calculation.

But there are additional reasons that are a little less obvious. First, firefighters keep their tools because the alternative of dropping them and using a shelter seems even riskier. The perceived risk is high largely because they have little familiarity with the alternative. Second, to drop one's tools is to admit failure; to keep one's tools is to reaffirm that one is still in, that the danger will pass, and that everything will work out. This rationale has a chilling resemblance to the insistence at the British Royal Infirmary[3] that the high number of fatalities in pediatric cardiac surgery was less than ideal but not unacceptably poor,[4] that help was on the way, that there was a potential for development,[5] that there was a run of bad luck,[6] and that the learning curve was slowed by an influx of complex cases. A third possibility is that people may hold on to their tools because of social dynamics. If a crew is lined up single file and marching up a trail, and if the first person in line keeps his or her tools, then the second person in line who sees this may conclude that the first person is not scared and feels no need for change. Having concluded that there is no cause for worry or that it would be too embarrassing to go back to camp as the only person without tools, the second person also retains his or her tools and is observed to do so by the third person in line, who similarly infers less danger than may exist. Each person individually may be fearful, but mistakenly conclude that everyone else is calm. Thus the situation appears to be safe, except no one actually believes that it is. The actions of the last person in line, the one who feels most intensely the fire nipping at his or her heels, is observed by no one, which means it is tough to convey the gravity of the situation back up the line. Thus, to the earlier, obvious reasons why people don't drop their tools we can now add the less obvious reasons of fear of unfamiliar technology, reluctance to admit failure in a can-do culture, and perception that fear is not widespread.

There is a third and final set of reasons that are even less obvious and may seem to border on the absurd. These are the very ones we need to linger over. There is evidence that some people at South Canyon didn't know how to drop their tools. Quentin Rhoades, who survived, describes running but being slowed because he was trying to find a place to put down his saw so it wouldn't be burned.[7] The same thing happened at Mann Gulch. In his testimony during the Mann Gulch accident investigation, Walter Rumsey mentioned that even though he was running for his life, he saw that Eldon Diettert was carrying a shovel. Rumsey grabbed it but then searched for a tree so he could carefully lean the shovel against it. People who have been trained to value and carry out whatever equipment they carry in to a fire might be at a disadvantage when, without any prior experience of what it feels like or how to do it, they are told to drop their tools.

It may seem odd to think that people keep their tools because they don't know how to drop them. But it is perhaps oddest of all to imagine that the firefighters didn't drop their tools because they didn't have any. But that's what I suspect happened. And that's what I suspect Berwick fears is happening in medical circles. Fire suppression and medical work call for capabilities that involve lives, people, even perhaps a calling. Firefighting tools such as the Pulaski are named after famous firefighters, they are designed solely for firefighting, and their skillful use is the mark of a seasoned firefighter and central to that person's identity. The fusion of tools with identities means that under conditions of threat it makes no more sense to drop one's tools than it does to drop one's pride or one's sense of self. Tools and identities form a unity without seams or separable elements.

Listen to Norman Maclean's reflections on firefighter identity at Mann Gulch:[8]

1. "When a firefighter is told to drop his firefighting tools, he is told to forget he is a firefighter and run for his life."[9]
2. "When firefighters are told to throw away their tools, they don't know who they are anymore, not even what gender."[10]

What is striking is the apparent *fusion* of tools with identities. When I first posed the question—Why don't firefighters drop their tools?—I assumed a separation between firefighters and tools that may not be their circumstance at all. Instead, their circumstance may be one of equipment, projects, and action in a context where there is no separation between subject and object. If that's true, then the detachment needed to separate people from their current dysfunctional tools may be concentrated in the younger generation of medical workers. There is evidence that novices are less likely than experts to fuse tools and identities and more likely to impose a subject-object separation on technology and procedures.[11] This leads to the unexpected prediction that those who die with their tools beside them may have more expertise than those who survive. Berwick's insistence that physicians and insurers decouple medical identity from office hours may be more plausible to novices and more readily adopted by them.

Berwick's treatment of his escape fire as an instance of "sensemaking" rather than decision making is reminiscent of a similar shift now occurring in wildland firefighting. Paul Gleason, reputed to be one of the five best wildland firefighters in the world, said that when he is fighting fires he prefers to view his leadership efforts as sensemaking rather than decision making. In his words, "If I make a decision it is a possession, I take pride in it, I tend to defend it and not listen to those who question it. If I make sense, then this is more dynamic and I listen and I can change it. A decision is something you polish. Sensemaking is a direction for the next period."[12] When Gleason perceives himself as making a decision, he reports that he postpones action so he can get the decision "right," and that after he makes the decision, he finds himself defending it rather than revising it to suit changing circumstances. Both polishing and defending eat up valuable time and encourage blind spots. If Gleason instead perceives himself as making sense of an unfolding fire, then he gives his crew a direction for some indefinite period, a direction that by definition is dynamic, open to revision at any time, self-correcting, and responsive, and more of its rationale is transparent. The presumption that medical decisions must be individual, infallible, and perfect draws attention away from the reality that you don't even know there is a decision to be made until you have first engaged in sensemaking. And in those acts of sensemaking are the interactions, the updating, the consultations, the trial and error, the listening, the reliance on systems, the wariness of fixation, the flexibility, and the safety that get ignored when a medical decision is lovingly polished and then arrogantly defended.

I think Berwick is right: Quality improvement is about escape fires and tools. But most of all it is about lightness: "In pursuit of knowledge, every day something is acquired; in pursuit of wisdom, every day something is dropped."[13]

Notes

1. Six died at the Dude fire, fourteen at South Canyon, two at the California fire, and one at the Buchanan fire. *Source:* Putnam, T. "Analysis of Escape Efforts and Personal Protective Equipment on the South Canyon Fire." *Wildfire*, 1995, 4(3), 42–47.

2. The Prineville Hotshots did not know Haugh, Erickson, Hipke, Thrash, or Roth, all five of whom were smokejumpers, and all five of whom told the hotshots either to run or to deploy shelters. Hotshots are trained to wait for orders from their own leaders. Six of the hotshots who died still had their fire shelters in their cases, presumably because no order had been given to deploy them. *Source:* Putnam, "Analysis of Escape Efforts and Personal Protective Equipment on the South Canyon Fire," 42–47.

3. Kennedy, I. *Learning from Bristol: The Report of the Public Inquiry into Children's Heart Surgery at Bristol Royal Infirmary, 1984–1995.* London: Her Majesty's Stationer, 2001.

4. Kennedy, *Learning from Bristol*, 163.

5. Kennedy, *Learning from Bristol*, 154.

6. Kennedy, *Learning from Bristol*, 248.

7. U.S. Forest Service. *Report of the South Canyon Fire Accident Investigation Team.* Washington, D.C.: August 17, 1994, A5–A69.

8. Maclean, N. *Young Men and Fire.* Chicago: University of Chicago Press, 1992.

9. Maclean, *Young Men and Fire*, 273.

10. Maclean, *Young Men and Fire*, 226.

11. Dreyfuss, H. L. "Intuitive, Deliberative, and Calculative Models of Expert Performance." In C. E. Zsambok and G. Klein (eds.), *Naturalistic Decision Making.* Mahwah, N.J.: Erlbaum, 1997, 17–28.

12. Personal communication, June 13, 1995.

13. Lao Tzu, cited in Muller, W. *Sabbath: Restoring the Sacred Rhythm of Rest.* New York: Bantam, 1999, 134.

Escape Fire

11th Annual National Forum on Quality Improvement in Health Care

New Orleans, Louisiana, December 7, 1999

These are the flowers of Mann Gulch (Figure 8.1).

And these are the markers of death (Figure 8.2).

Twenty miles north of Helena, Montana, the Missouri River flowing north cuts into the eastern slope of the Rocky Mountains on the first leg of its great, semicircular, 2,500-mile journey to

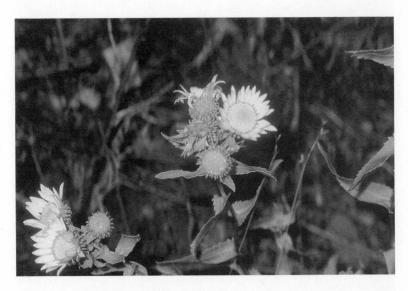

Figure 8.1. The Flowers of Mann Gulch.
Source: Photo by Paul B. Batalden.

Keynote speech presented at 11th Annual National Forum on Quality Improvement in Health Care, New Orleans, Louisiana, December 7, 1999.

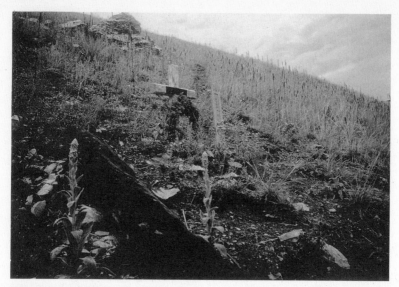

Figure 8.2. The Markers of Death.
Source: Photo by Paul B. Batalden.

meet the Mississippi. Lewis and Clark passed through this spec-
tacular formation on July 19, 1805, and named it "Gates of the
Mountains." Two miles downriver from the Gates, a small, two-
mile-long canyon runs down to the Missouri from the northeast.
This is Mann Gulch.

It is the site of a tragedy: the Mann Gulch fire (Figure 8.3). More
than fifty years ago, on August 5, 1949, thirteen young men—twelve
smokejumpers and one fireguard with the U.S. Forest Service—lost
their lives here in a fire that did not behave as they expected it to.
Although the disaster, the first one in which smokejumpers died,
was headline news at the time, the story fell into relative obscurity
until a book appeared. Called *Young Men and Fire*, it was written by
Norman Maclean, a Shakespeare scholar and the author of *A River
Runs Through It*. Maclean, who had fought forest fires as a young
man, became obsessed with the Mann Gulch story and spent two
decades researching it. His book was published in 1992, two years
after his death at age eighty-seven.

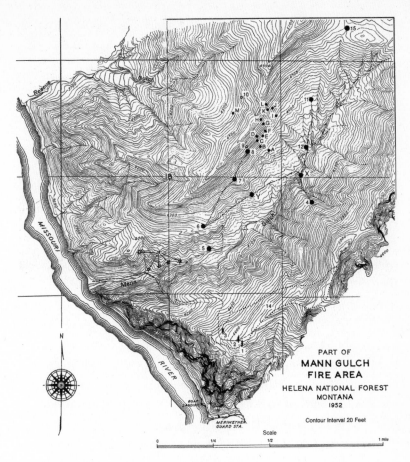

Figure 8.3. Map of Mann Gulch Fire Area.
Source: Used by persmission of USDA Forest Service.

Many of you have probably read *Young Men and Fire*. For those who haven't, let me briefly tell the story.

On the afternoon of August 4, 1949, a lightning storm started a small fire near the top of the southeast ridge of Mann Gulch—Meriwether Ridge, a slope forested with Douglas fir and ponderosa pine. The fire was spotted the next day; by 2:30 P.M., a C-47 transport plane had flown out of Missoula, Montana, carrying sixteen smokejumpers. One got sick and didn't jump. The rest—fifteen men between seventeen and thirty-three years old—parachuted to the head of the gulch at 4:10 P.M. Their radio didn't make it. Its chute failed to open and it crashed. They were joined on the ground by a fireguard, who had spotted the fire. Otherwise, the smokejumpers were isolated from the outside world.

The smokejumpers were a new organization, barely nine years old in 1949. Building in part on military experience from World War II, they were reinventing the approach to forest fire containment—aggressive, highly tactical, and coordinated. To them, the Mann Gulch fire, covering sixty acres at the time of the jump, appeared routine. It was what they called a "ten o'clock fire," meaning they would have it beaten by ten o'clock in the morning of the day after they jumped.

They were wrong.

The first reconnaissance team headed down the south side of the gulch. The foreman, Wag Dodge, became worried that the group could get trapped on that side. He ordered them to come back and cross with the rest of the men to the north side of the gulch, opposite the fire, and head down the hill so that the river, an escape route, would be at their backs as they fought the fire.

The north side of the gulch was grassland, covered in bunchgrass thirty inches tall, with almost no trees. It was unfamiliar terrain to these firefighters, who had been trained in the forests around Missoula.

Dodge was the first to spot the impending disaster—the fire had jumped the gulch from the south side to the north. It had ignited the grass only two hundred yards ahead of the lead smokejumpers, blocking their route to the river. No one had seen the potential for this flanking action because the downhill view was obstructed by a series of low ridges and they had no detailed maps.

Now a race began. Dodge knew that the grassfire would cut off the route to the river and would head swiftly up the north slope toward the firefighters. He ordered the group to reverse course immediately and head back up the slope toward the ridge crest, hoping to get over it before the fire did.

The north slope of Mann Gulch is steep—a 76 percent slope on the average. Photos don't capture the reality. You have to go there to understand. It is hard even to walk up such a slope, but these young men were trying to run up it. Add air one hundred degrees at the start and superheated by the rushing fire, add the poor visibility from smoke and airborne debris, add the weight of the packs and tools these men were taught never to drop, and add their inexperience with the pace and heat of grassfires—far hotter and moving a lot faster than fires in forests. At 5:45 P.M., when the crew turned around, the fire was traveling toward them at 120 feet per minute, or 1.4 miles an hour. Ten minutes later, at 5:55 P.M., it was traveling at 610 feet per minute—7 miles an hour.

Wag Dodge knew they would lose the race to the top. With the fire barely two hundred yards behind him, he did a strange and marvelous thing. He invented a solution. On the spot. His crew must have thought he had gone crazy as he took some matches out of his pocket, bent down, lit a match, and set fire to the grass directly in front of him. The new fire spread quickly uphill ahead of him and he stepped into the middle of the newly burnt area. He called to his crew to join him as he lay down in the middle of the burnt ground. Dodge had invented what is now called an "escape fire," and soon after Mann Gulch it became a standard part of the training of all Forest Service firefighters.

But on August 5, 1949, no one followed Wag Dodge. They ignored him, or they didn't hear him, and they ran right past the answer. The fire raged past Wag Dodge and overtook the crew. Only three made it to the top of the ridge, and one of the three was so badly burned that he died a few hours later. Of the sixteen men who had fought the fire, three lived: Robert Sallee and Walter Rumsey, who made it over the crest, and Wag Dodge, who survived nearly unharmed in his escape fire.

When I first read *Young Men and Fire*, the story gripped me. I didn't understand why until I read a paper by Professor Karl E. Weick of the University of Michigan. Weick is a student of organizations, especially organizations under stress, and even more especially, organizations that are able to function well under trying conditions, the so-called high-reliability organizations, such as aircraft carriers and the smokejumpers at their best. His paper is called "The Collapse of Sensemaking in Organizations: The Mann Gulch Disaster." I want to review some of Weick's main points here, and then I will find my way—though you probably think I can't—back to health care.

Weick asks two questions about the Mann Gulch tragedy: Why did the smokejumpers' organization unravel? And how can such organizations be made more resilient?

Weick regards the group of Mann Gulch smokejumpers as an organization and he thinks that one of the key roles of organizations is what he calls *sensemaking*. He has written a fine book called *Sensemaking in Organizations*. Sensemaking is the process through which the fluid, multilayered world is given order, within which people can orient themselves, find purpose, and take effective action. Weick is a postmodern thinker. He believes that there is little or no preexisting sense of organization in the world—that is, no order that comes before the definition of order. Organizations don't discover sense, they create it.

Weick tells the story of a reconnaissance group of soldiers lost in the Alps on a training mission. It was winter, they had no maps, and they seemed hopelessly lost. They were preparing to die when one soldier found a map crushed down at the bottom of his pack. With the map in hand they regained their courage, bivouacked for the night, and proceeded out of the mountains the next day to rescue. Only when they were recuperating in the main camp did someone notice that the map they had been using wasn't a map of the Alps at all; it was a map of the Pyrenees. Weick uses this story to point out that sensemaking is an act of its own, valuable in itself, and independent of any notion of reality. "This story raises the remarkable idea," he says, "that, when you are lost, any map will do."

In groups of interdependent people, organizations create sense out of possible chaos. Organizations unravel when sensemaking collapses, when they can no longer supply meaning, when they cling to interpretations that no longer work.

For the Mann Gulch smokejumpers, what appeared to be a small, manageable fire quickly turned into something unknown, and much more dangerous. Weick calls this sudden loss of meaning a *cosmology episode*. The experience is fundamental and terrifying— the group, the roles, the interrelationships, the tools, the orderliness that the sensemaking organization had provided collapse and people are left alone, unable to communicate with one another. They panic.

Weick supplies a "recipe" for the collapse of sensemaking: "Thrust people into unfamiliar roles; leave some key roles unfilled; make the task more ambiguous; discredit the role system; and make all of these changes in a context in which small things can combine into something monstrous." Now maybe my route back to health care is becoming a little bit clearer.

Is health care unraveling? Are we in a cosmology episode?

In a recent survey of forty-two medical group practices about morale among physicians and office staff, only 15 percent of the respondents rated their work environment as good or excellent. Medicare and Medicaid managed care rolls are dropping monthly. We have tens of millions of uninsured Americans, significant medication errors in seven out of every one hundred inpatients, tenfold or more variation in population-based rates of important surgical procedures, 30 percent overuse of advanced antibiotics, excessive waits throughout our system of care, 50 percent or more underuse of effective and inexpensive medications for heart attacks and immunization for the elderly, and declining service ratings from patients and their families. In 1998, the American Customer Satisfaction Index rated Americans' satisfaction with hospitals at 70 percent, just below the U.S. Postal Service (71 percent) and just above the Internal Revenue Service (69 percent). Racial gaps in health status remain enormous; a black male born in Baltimore today will on average live eight years less than an average white male. All this happens with per capita health care costs 30 to 40 percent higher in the United States than in the next most expensive nation.

But is the health care system unraveling? Isn't that going a bit too far?

I face a personal dilemma here. This has been a tough year for my family, especially for my wife, Ann, who last spring began developing symptoms of a rare and serious autoimmune spinal cord problem. In early March, Ann competed in a twenty-eight-kilometer cross-country ski race in Alaska. Two months later she couldn't walk across our bedroom. From April through September Ann had six hospitalizations for a total of more than sixty inpatient days in three institutions, while she gradually experienced increasing pain, lost the ability to walk, and became essentially bedridden. For most of that time, nobody could tell us exactly what was happening or what her prognosis was. I can report some better news now, because Ann has clearly begun to improve. She can now walk long distances with a cane, she is beginning to get back to her work, and she and I think she is going to be all right, though it will take a long time.

My dilemma is this: Our ordeal has been enormously painful and intensely private, and it is by no means over yet. To use it for any public purpose, even to speak about it, risks crossing a boundary of propriety and confidentiality that ought not to be crossed. Yet this has been the formative experience for me overall in the past year— the experience of the decade—and it resonates so thoroughly with the mission of improving health care that not to learn from it also seems wrong.

I asked Ann for permission to speak about her illness and she agreed. She and I both hope that some good can come of it.

Let me first say that this painful summer and fall has left me more impressed than I have ever been with the goodwill, kindness, generosity, commitment, and dignity of the people who work in health care—almost all of them. Day after day and night after night, Ann, our children, and I have been deeply touched by acts of consideration, empathy, and technical expertise that these good people—nurses, doctors, technicians, housekeepers, dieticians, volunteers, and aides of all sorts—have brought to her bedside. The kindness crosses all boundaries. I asked Ann what she regards as the most impressive moments of help in her inpatient experience, and she mentioned first a housekeeper who every evening would come into her room and, while cleaning, talk about her children and ours—a common humanity. Ann also remembers the young infectious-disease fellow who, in the darkest of our hours, sat by Ann's bed and said what we were feeling: "Not knowing is the worst thing of all." Until then, no one had quite labeled this deep source of suffering.

For these incessant kindnesses we are deeply grateful. We were fortunate indeed to have access to care in several of the finest hospitals in our nation.

Which makes it hard to tell the other side of the story too. Put very, very simply: the people work well, by and large, but the system often does not. Every hour of our care reminded me, and alerted Ann, about the enormous, costly, and painful gaps between what we got in our days of need and what we needed. The experience did not actually surprise me, but it did shock me. Put in other terms, as a friend of mine said, before this I was concerned; now, I am radicalized. If what happened to Ann could happen in our best institutions, I wonder more than ever before what the average must be like.

Above all we needed safety, yet Ann was unsafe. I have read the work of physician Lucian Leape that documents medication errors, but now I have seen them firsthand, at the sharp end, sitting by Ann's bedside for week after week of acute care. The errors were not rare; they were the norm. During one admission, the neurologist told us in the morning, "By no means should you be getting anticholinergic agents," and a medication with profound anti-cholinergic side effects was given that afternoon. The attending neurologist in another admission told us by phone that a crucial and potentially toxic drug should be started immediately. He said, "Time is of the essence." That was on Thursday morning at 10:00 A.M. The first dose was given sixty hours later—on Saturday night at 10:00 P.M. Nothing I could do, nothing I did, nothing I could think of made any difference. It nearly drove me mad. Colace was discontinued by a physician's order on day one, and was nonetheless brought by the nurse every single evening throughout a fourteen-day admission. Ann was supposed to receive five intravenous doses of a very toxic chemotherapy agent, but dose three was labeled as dose two. For half a day no record could be found that dose two had ever been given, even though I had watched it drip in myself. I tell you from my personal observation: no day passed—not one—without a medication error. Most weren't serious, but they scared us.

We needed consistent, reliable information, based, we would have hoped, on the best science available. Instead we often heard a cacophony of meaningless and sometimes contradictory conclusions. Ann received Cytoxan, which causes hair loss and low white blood cell count. *When would these occur?* we asked. The answers varied by a factor of five. Drugs tried and proven futile in one admission would be recommended in the next as if they were fresh ideas. A spinal tap was done for a test for Lyme disease, but the doctor collected too little fluid for the test and the tap had to be repeated. During a crucial phase of diagnosis, one doctor told us to hope that the diagnosis would be of a certain disease, because that disease has a benign course. That same evening, another doctor told us to hope for the opposite, because that same disease is relentless—sometimes fatal. Complex, serial information on blood counts, temperature, functional status, and weight—the information on the basis of which risky and expensive decisions were relying—was collected in disorganized, narrative formats, embedded in nursing notes and daily forms. As far as I know, the only person who ever drew a graph of

Ann's fevers or white blood cell counts was me, and the data were so complex and crossed so many settings that, short of a graph, no rational interpretation was possible. As a result, physicians often reached erroneous conclusions, such as assuming that Ann had improved after a specific treatment when in fact she had improved before it, or not at all. The experience of patienthood, or patient-spousehood, as the case may be, was often one of trying to get the attention of decision makers to correct their impressions or assumptions. Sociologically, this proved very tough, as we felt time and again our migration to the edge of the label "difficult patient."

We needed respect for our privacy, personal attention, and timely care. Often we got it. But often we didn't. On at least three occasions Ann waited alone for over an hour, cold and frightened on a gurney in the waiting area outside an MRI unit in a subbasement in the middle of the night. A nurse insisted that Ann swallow her pills while she watched, "because elderly patients sometimes drop their medicines." Ann's bedtime was 10:00 P.M., but her sleeping medication was often brought at 8:00 P.M., to accommodate changes in nursing shifts. By day thirty of hospitalization, Ann knew exactly which sleeping pills would work and which would not, yet it was a daily struggle to get the right ones to her, as new clinicians insisted on trying their own approaches, ignoring Ann's expertise. One place gave a sleeping pill at 3:00 A.M., and then routinely woke Ann at 4:00 A.M. to take her blood pressure, which never varied from normal. An emergency room visit for a diagnostic spinal tap that should have taken two hours evolved into an eleven-hour ordeal of constant delay.

In all of our hospitalizations there have been only two instances when someone sought our feedback on the care system itself. Only two people ever asked us to make suggestions about how their system could be improved.

We needed continuity. Ann's story was extremely complex and evolved over many weeks. Yet we often felt that the only real memories in the system were ours. Times of transition of responsibility, such as the first of the month, were especially trying. On one first of the month the new senior attending physician walked into Ann's room, cheerfully introduced himself, and asked, "So how long have you had MS?" Ann doesn't have MS. Over and over and over again Ann had to tell her story, which became longer and more complex as time passed. By the fifth or tenth or fifteenth iteration, that there was any plausibility to the common explanation—"fresh minds, two heads are better than one"—gave way to our doubts that any of these caring people ever talked to one another at all. "Discharge" from a hospital really meant it. I would estimate that fifty different doctors and three times as many nurses became closely— intensely—involved with Ann's care in hospitals. Yet to my knowledge only three of these individuals made any effort to follow Ann's course after any particular discharge, and these three are actively managing Ann's outpatient care at this time. The rest have, I suspect, no way at all to know how she is faring, or whether their diagnoses and prognoses were, after all, correct. Continuity, when it occurred, was based on acts of near heroism. Ann's primary neurologist travels frequently for speaking engagements. When he was away during crucial times, he phoned Ann every day, whether from Amsterdam, London, Geneva, or San Francisco.

One after another, caregivers told us of their own distress. The occupational therapist (OT) apologized for cutting back Ann's treatment, explaining that seventeen OTs had been laid off the week before. The doctors told us about insurance forms and fights for needed hospital days. The nurses complained that the transport service never came.

And the bills were astounding. They have been covered by our insurance, for which we are immensely grateful. But I cannot reconcile what happened with the fees—for example, pharmacy charges of $30 for a single pill. Remember the Colace that was discontinued but brought anyway? Well, there it is: pill by pill, charges for all the days on which the nurse opened the unneeded packet and threw it in the garbage. Radiology charges of $155 per film for second readings of fourteen films transferred from one hospital to another. MRI scans over and over again for $1,700, $2,000, $2,200 per procedure. Ann's care has been billed at perhaps $150,000 so far, at a minimum, and the bare fact is that of all that enormous investment, a remarkably small percentage—half at best, probably much less—stood any chance at all of helping her. The rest has been pure waste. Even while simpler needs—for a question answered, information explained, a word of encouragement, or just good and nourishing food—have gone unmet.

Not all of these flaws in care were equally present in all of the hospitals. Some hospitals were much better than others. In fact, if we could combine the best of care in each, we would have a system far closer to ideal. But some of these defects existed everywhere, and this was in some of the best hospitals in America.

I am deeply, deeply grateful for the people, and I respect the institutions a great deal. But we have so much left to do. We are causing harm and we need to stop it. I think the fire has jumped the gulch. The blaze is on our side. As I waited helplessly for Ann to get a medicine when time was "of the essence," I even felt the fire licking at my heels.

The people know this. Not just the people in the beds, but the people doing the work too. The doctors and nurses and technicians and managers and pharmacists and all the rest know—*they must know*—the truth. They see it every day, and even if their defensive routines no longer permit them to say what they see, they do see it: errors, delays, nonsensical variation, lack of communication, misinformation, the care environment not at all a place of healing.

"Why do organizations unravel?" asks Karl Weick. "Because they no longer make sense of the world," he answers. I love medicine. I love the purpose of our work. But we are unraveling, I think. Sense is collapsing.

Yet this does not need to happen. Sensemaking is within our reach. Karl Weick asks a second question, with much more embedded optimism: "How can organizations be made more resilient?"

He answers that resilience has four sources in organizations, equipping them to, in his words, "forestall deterioration" of their sensemaking function.

First, there is *improvisation*, the ability to invent when old formulas fail. The young men at Mann Gulch had been trained to never, under any circumstances, drop their tools. One of their tools was a Pulaski, a combination axe and pick that is very useful in fighting forest fires. It's not useful to carry it up a 76 percent slope when a grassfire is racing toward you at 610 feet per minute. Yet the reconstructed journeys of the victims of the fire show that several carried their Pulaskis a good way up the hill as they raced for their lives. Wag Dodge, in the midst of ultimate crisis, improvised the escape fire, though no one followed him.

Second, there are what Weick calls *virtual role systems*. These systems refer to the ability of individuals to carry, as it were, a social system inside their heads—to assume structures even when they are not externally apparent. If the smokejumper crew had still seen Wag Dodge as their leader when he invented his escape fire, maybe they would have followed him. They didn't: the smoke and fear and noise and shock had not only disrupted the smokejumper system as a formal entity, but it had also disrupted its representation in the mind of each individual. The organization could have been preserved if individual minds had held on to it, but they did not. The system fragmented and the roles disappeared.

Third, says Weick, resilience within an organization is maintained by *the attitude of wisdom*. He quotes John Meacham, who writes, "Ignorance and knowledge grow together. . . . To be wise is not to know particular facts but to know without excessive confidence or excessive cautiousness. . . . [In changing times] organizations most need . . . curiosity, openness, and complex sensing."

Fourth and finally, Weick says, resilience requires *respectful interaction*. "If a role system collapses among people for whom trust, honesty, and self-respect are underdeveloped," Weick maintains, "then they are on their own. And fear often swamps their resourcefulness. If, however, a role system collapses among people where trust, honesty, and self-respect are more fully developed, then new options . . . are created."

I think that this idea—the loss of sensemaking—is a powerful vocabulary for interpreting the health care crisis of our time. At least it captures the most disturbing aspects of what Ann and I experienced this year. If I'm right, then it might lead us to new ideas that are every bit as tough to embrace as Wag Dodge's escape fire, and every bit as promising. I want to imagine health care's escape fire, and I want to be bold.

I have decided to divide the question into two parts. It seems to me that the health care system's capacity to preserve sensemaking in a time of crisis requires change at two levels. I call them preconditions and designs.

Preconditions are a set of shared assumptions that don't tell us what future we need to build but give us a chance of staying in order long enough to tackle that issue. They make sense possible.

Designs are the basic ideas behind the escape fire itself. They are the new ways of thinking about what we do. The new sense. The scheme we create together to organize a world that threatens otherwise to become chaotic and overtake us.

I can see five preconditions that give us a chance at sensemaking.

The first is the toughest: *We need to face reality.* This is very, very hard. Why did it take the Mann Gulch crew so long to realize they were in trouble? The soundest explanation is not that the threat was too small to see; it is that it was too big. Some problems are too overwhelming to name. I now think that that is where we have come in health care; I *have* been radicalized. Our challenge is not to develop more sensitive ways to detect our risks, our errors, our flaws, our variation, our indignities, our fragmentation, our delays, our waste, our insults to the people we say we exist to serve. Our challenge is to have the courage to name clearly and boldly the problems we have—many—and their size—immense. We must find ways to do this without either marginalizing the truth-teller or demoralizing the good people working in these bad systems.

David Lawrence, former CEO of Kaiser Permanente Foundation Health Plan, has said it best: "The chassis is broken." Our challenges are not marginal and their solutions are not incremental. The sooner we get honest about those facts, the sooner we can get on with the job.

The second precondition is that we need to *drop the Pulaskis*. Our current tools can't do the job. We can't get where we need to go by stressing the current system. We can't possibly run fast enough up a 76 percent slope.

Let me show you the difference. At the Institute for Healthcare Improvement, we have two bathrooms. Each has a sign on the door that can be set in two positions: vacant or occupied (Figure 8.4). You flip the sign as you enter and leave. Or you don't. In seventy-one observations, I obtained the following data. The sign was correct forty-three out of seventy-one times, or 61 percent of the time.

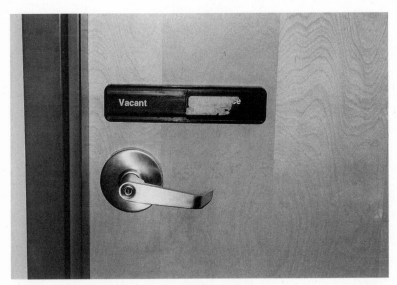

Figure 8.4. Bathroom Door with Vacancy Sign.

It was wrong 39 percent of the time. The most common error, 30 percent of the time, was that the sign said "occupied" when the room was actually vacant. This error causes moderate to severe discomfort in timid staff members who do not check the door handle. The other error, 10 percent of the time, was that the sign said "vacant" when the room was actually occupied. This error can cause injury if a staff member tries to pull the door and it is locked, or embarrassment if he or she trusts the sign and the occupant has forgotten to lock the door.

The sign system functions poorly. In fact, if you simply guessed that the room was vacant, you would have been right forty-four times out of seventy-one, or 62 percent of the time—more often than the sign.

I decided to fix the system by emphasizing it. Here is my reminder sign (Figure 8.5). It never lasted more than an hour before someone tore it down. I tried to highlight its importance by making a sign for the sign for the sign (Figure 8.6), but that too was torn

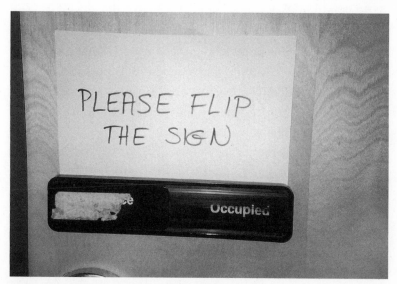

Figure 8.5. Bathroom Door with Reminder Sign.

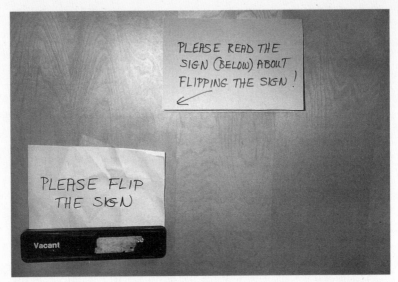

Figure 8.6. Bathroom Door with Reminder Sign About Reminder Sign.

down. The experiment ended with a surge of graffiti, which I thought lacked taste.

Such an approach will never work. On the other hand, you and I have both been in airplanes with a lavatory sign system that is right nearly 100 percent of the time. The reason is that the locking system in airplane lavatories uses a design principle called a "forcing function." It doesn't allow for choice—you can't lock the door or turn on the light without changing the sign, and you can't open the door without changing the sign again.

Our health care escape fire will have the same principles. It will not just invoke different tools, it will force us to drop the old ones. Health care's backpack is full of useless assumptions that are so old and so often repeated that they have become wisdom from the mouth of Hippocrates himself, and one questions them at grave risk to one's professional relationships.

Precondition number three is that we *stay in formation*. Weick refers to this as having virtual role models. In the Mann Gulch fire, the organization disappeared at the moment of crisis. It became every man for himself. Nobody remembered that Wag Dodge was the most experienced and the leader, or that together the crew might learn something that separately they could not. The men's bodies afterward were literally strewn for three hundred yards across the slope.

Successful sensemaking can't leave anyone out. Health care's disintegration is not yet every man for himself, but it is every discipline for itself, every guild for itself. As a result we tend to assume today that one guild's solution cannot be another's. We assume that either we will preserve quality or cut costs; that patients will get what they ask for or science will prevail; that managers will run the show or doctors will be in control; that the bottom line is financial or moral.

This won't work. No comprehensive solution is possible if it fails to make sense to any of the key stakeholders. At least four parts of our crew need to share in the solution—a common answer—or the crew will fall apart. Whatever escape fire we create has to make sense in the world of science and professionalism, in the world of the patient and family, in the world of the business and finance of health care, and in the world of the good, kind people who do the work of caring. I think the toughest part of this may be in terms of the business and financing of care. There is a tendency to assume that financial success—as in thriving organizations—and great care are mutually exclusive. We will not make progress, however, unless and until these goals become aligned with each other.

The fourth precondition is procedural: to achieve sense, we have to *talk to one another, and listen*. Sensemaking is fundamentally an enterprise of interdependency, and the currency of interdependency is conversation. In the noise and smoke of the fire, just when our interdependency is most crucial, it becomes most difficult to communicate. This will not do. Civil, open dialogue is a precondition for success.

The fifth and final precondition for success is *leadership*. You don't achieve sense without having leaders. Effective leaders in high-reliability organizations exhibit certain skills: clearly defining tasks, demonstrating their own competence, disavowing perfection so as to encourage openness, and engaging and building the team. Leadership like this makes constructive, informed interactions more likely, and at a deeper level, leaves the sensemaking apparatus intact as the context changes.

I believe that these five preconditions—facing reality, dropping the old tools, staying in formation, communicating, and having capable leadership—set the stage for making sense as the fire blows up. Now we have a chance. What does the escape fire look like?

I think that health care's escape fire has three primary design elements. None is totally new, but together, fully realized, they would create a care system that is as different from today's as a 76 percent slope is from an escape fire. I will call these elements *access*, *science*, and *relationships*.

Access is the property of a system that promises, "We are there for you." The current system of care is embedded with processes and assumptions that ration, limit, and control access. To get help requires appointments, permission, authorization, waiting, forms, and procedures to which the person in need must bend his or her need. In the current system, *first* we allocate the supply, and *then* we experience the demand. We accept as inevitable that accessibility at some times—weekends, nights, holidays—is of course different from what it is from nine to five. Demand often feels unpredictable, threatening, and even hostile, and we reply with equal unpredictability, threat, and counteraccusations about insatiable patients and unrealistic expectations.

All of this changes in the escape fire. The new system of access can be summarized this way: 24/7/365. The access to help that we will envision is uncompromising, meeting whatever need exists, whenever and wherever it exists, in whatever form is requested.

Before the howling starts let me remind you of one precondition: Drop your Pulaskis. With the current tools, 24/7/365 is not at all achievable. Meeting demand this well within current frameworks is harder than running a marathon up a 76 percent grade. It cannot be done.

Our Pulaski in the search for access is the encounter—the visit. Total access 24/7/365 begins to be achievable only when we—scientists, professionals, patients, payers, and the health care workforce—agree that the product we choose to make is not visits. Our product is healing relationships, and these can be fashioned in many new and wonderful forms if we suspend the old ways of making sense of care.

The access we need to create is access to help and healing, and that does not always mean—in fact, I think it rarely means—reliance on face-to-face meetings between patients, doctors, and nurses. Tackled well, I believe, this new framework will gradually reveal that half or more of our encounters—maybe as many as 80 percent of them—are neither wanted by patients nor deeply believed in by professionals. This is an example of a problem so big that we have trouble seeing it. The health care encounter as a face-to-face visit is a dinosaur. More exactly, it is a form of relationship of immense and irreplaceable value to a few of the people we seek to help, and these few have their access severely curtailed by the use of visits to meet the needs of the many whose needs could be better met through other kinds of encounters.

The alternatives to visits in the escape fire are many: self-care strongly supported and unequivocally encouraged; group visits of patients with like needs with or without professionals involved; Internet use for access to scientific and popular information; e-mail care between patients and clinicians; and well-managed chat rooms, electronic and real, for patients and significant others who face common challenges.

Payers should take careful note: most of you still pay only for Pulaskis. The greatest potential for reducing costs while maintaining and improving the lot of patients is to replace visits with better, more flexible, and fine-tuned forms of care. But almost all current payment mechanisms, whether enforced by the market or mapped into organizations by internal compensation systems, use impoverished definitions of productivity that discourage the search for and incorporation of nonvisit care.

Another form of access is access to one's own medical information; this too is a form of nonvisit care. An employee of the Institute for Healthcare Improvement recently had a test done for a potentially serious disease. She called the clinical office for the result and heard the following: "Yes, Ms. Smith, . . . your result is right here. It is . . . uh-oh . . . ah . . . Ms. Smith, I am not authorized to give you this information. You will need to talk with the doctor. He will be back tomorrow." When my wife was on Cytoxan, she and I were the only people who were actually tracking her white blood cell count graphically, yet several of her nurses refused to tell us the white cell count results when they became available.

The medical record properly belongs to the patient, not to the care system. It must become an open book to the patient, available without restriction, hesitation, or suspicion. Diane Plamping, a public health researcher from the United Kingdom, offered me the following rule about access to information: "Nothing about me without me."

In my escape fire we will have a new view of the nature of information in health care. In the current model, information is treated generally as a tool for retrospection, a record of what has happened, a stable asset that we may or may not use to recall the past or to defend or prosecute a lawsuit.

Here in my escape fire, the view of information is different. Information, we now see, *is* care. People want knowledge, and the transfer of knowledge is caring itself. Whenever we put a block or bottleneck in the way of knowledge transfer—whether we call it an appointment or permission or even a decision by anyone other than the person who wants to know—we add cost without value and fail to meet need. We also put 24/7/365 even further from our reach.

I recently visited a magnificent new hospital that has developed a state-of-the-art health information library for patients. There were computer terminals everywhere, user-friendly books, three-dimensional models, and a full collection of instructional video-tapes. I spoke to the nurse who ran the library and she complained that it was vastly underutilized because they were having a hard time getting doctors to send their patients there.

I asked, "Why not go directly to the patients and get the doctors out of the loop?"

She said, "The doctors would never go for that."

I wanted to say, "Come into my escape fire. In here we know that information is a form of care, and that doctors' visits and decisions are too. And we want to make sure that anyone who needs either gets it. Doctors are useful for some forms of caring; information resources like yours are useful for others."

So, the first element of my escape fire is *total access, without compromise: 24/7/365*.

The second element is *science*. At its best, the help we offer is based in knowledge. When care matches knowledge, it is most reliable. When care does not match knowledge, we fail to help, either by omission (failing to do what would help) or by waste (doing what cannot help). The current world is far too tolerant of mismatches between knowledge and action, far too permissive with omission and waste. As a result, our care is unreliable, our answers are inconsistent, and our practices vary without sense.

The escape fire looks different. I urge here that we adopt my colleague Dr. James Reinertsen's formulation, "All and only": "We will promise to deliver, reliably and without error, *all* the care that will help, and *only* the care that will help."

The Pulaski here may be an illogical commitment to the autonomy of clinical decisions. Just as the hospital with the patients' library illogically places the doctor between the patient and the information the patient wants, so the system fundamentally committed to autonomy places the individual doctor's mind between the patient and the best knowledge anywhere. Doctor visits are irreplaceable, sometimes; so is a doctor's autonomy to ensure that the patient is well served. But in my escape fire I would place a commitment to excellence—standardization to the best-known method—above clinician autonomy as a rule for care.

Physicians stand only to gain from this change of perspective. They know, as I do, that the volume of scientific medical literature today far outpaces the capacity of any one doctor—any one hundred doctors—to stay up to date. Dr. Larry Weed—a physician and specialist in medical informatics—says that asking an individual doctor to rely on his memory to store and retrieve all the facts relevant to patient care is like asking travel agents to memorize airline schedules. The art of the physician is to synthesize many different sources of information; this art should be used exactly and only when less expensive, less creative resources will not suffice.

This issue does not begin with a commitment to artificial intelligence or knowledge management. It begins with a commitment to excellence as the standard.

This includes a commitment to safety for patients and for staff. By some calculations, the aviation industry's safety record is better than health care's by a factor of one thousand or more. And aviation safety has improved tenfold in the past three decades, during a period of massive growth in volume and technology. This has been accomplished through science, not through exhortation. There are safe designs and there are unsafe designs. The issue has very little to do with the will or capability of human beings, who almost never intend errors to happen. It has a lot to do with whether leaders, board members, and managers employ the best available knowledge about safe designs for tasks, equipment, rules, and environments instead of relying on outmoded traditions and impoverished theories about motivation and "trying harder."

A scientific system of care would guarantee that the best-known approach is the standard approach.

The third element of the escape fire I will call *relationships* or, perhaps, *interactions*. While the first element, access, encourages us to consider how people get to the help they need, and the second element, science, asks us to consider how we can ensure that the best knowledge informs action, the interactions element challenges our current notions of the very nature of help itself. It raises the question of what, in the end, we are spending $1 trillion to produce. It is about our purposes.

In Mann Gulch, the transition of purpose was stark and total—from defeating a ten o'clock fire to saving lives. Until that event, the smokejumpers' training and intent were focused almost entirely on the first task and very little on the second. They felt invincible. After Mann Gulch it became clear to all that smokejumper safety and survival was a task on its own, and the most important one.

In the current framework, health care tends to regard human interaction more as a toll or price than as a goal or product. The system tends to act as if interactions were the burden it must bear so it can deliver the care. As a result, behaviors and systems emerge to control or limit interactions—as if they were a form of waste—and to regard commitment to interaction as a secondary issue in training, resource allocation, hiring, firing, and incentive.

In the escape fire, we see it differently. Here we know that interaction is not the price of care; it is care itself. A patient with a question presents an opportunity, not a burden. Time spent in building patients' skills in self-care is not a way to shift care; it *is* care. Access to information is desirable not because it improves care or supports compliance, but because it is a form of care.

University of Michigan education professor David Cohen says that no education occurs until what he calls "inert" assets (books, teachers, rooms, curricula, rules, budgets, and so on) interact with each other and with students. Education is interaction. People in educational organizations, he says, often behave as if the inert assets were essential and the interactions expendable. They fight political wars over budgets, space, and personnel, and spend little time defending and perfecting the interactions among these assets through cooperation, communication, teamwork, and knowledge about students.

It is the same in health care. Care is not doctors, nurses, hospitals, computers, books, rules, or medicines. These are inert. Care is interaction among our assets and between assets and patients. To perfect care, we must perfect interactions.

Four properties of interaction ought to be objects of investment and continual improvement in the escape fire. The first we have already covered: *to regard information transfer as a key form of care and to increase the accessibility, openness, reliability, and completeness of information for patients and families*. Generic, scientific, and patient information should be available to them without restriction or delay. "Nothing about me without me" is a formula for idealized interaction just as it is for idealized access.

Second, *interactions should be tailored to patients' needs*. The call to arms here comes to me from a friend named Art Berarducci, who, when he was CEO of a small hospital, placed over the entrance a sign that read, "Every patient is the only patient." Each person in need brings to us a unique set of qualities that require unique responses. The overall list of such qualities may be familiar: comfort, dignity, communication, privacy, involvement of loved ones, respect for cultural and ethnic differences, need for control and sharing in decisions, and so on. But for each individual, "quality of care" means balancing these various needs at levels that only the individual patient can determine. In the escape fire, we are not finished—we have not achieved excellence—until each individual is well served according to his or her needs, not ours. Our measure of successful interaction is not just an average of how we have done in the past for "them," but the answer to the inquiry, How did I just do for you?

Third, interactions in the escape fire begin with this assumption: *The patient is the source of all control*. We act only when the patient grants that privilege, each time. The current system—the one ablaze—often behaves as if control over decisions, resources, access, and information begins in the hands of the caregivers and is only ceded to patients when the caregivers choose to do so.

My wife had a surgical procedure and awoke in the recovery room asking for me. I was not permitted to join her for almost ninety minutes, even though she repeatedly asked that I be allowed to comfort her. Why did that staff and that institution willfully separate a man and his wife at a time when they could have offered support to one another? By what right does a nurse, doctor, or manager make a decision that violates basic principles of human decency and caring? As a husband and as a physician, I know that the rationale for asserting that right stands on infirm ground. In any other setting, such an act would obviously be wrong. In this setting, it is less obvious, but it is still wrong.

Control begins in the hands of the people we serve. If we caregivers wish to take it, we must ask. If a patient denies control, then we must accept their will as a matter of right. We are not hosts in our organizations so much as we are guests in our patients' lives.

Finally, *the interactions we nurture should be transparent.* People often say that health care needs more accountability. I have never quite known what that means. But I do understand the notion of transparency, and why it may help in the sensemaking process and perhaps better achieve what those who urge accountability mean. In the old world, burning now, there is a premium on secrecy. The highly desirable goal of confidentiality has mutated into a monstrous system of closed doors and locked cabinets. "Nothing about me without me" has a necessary correlate: "I can discover what affects me." Health care should be confidential, but the health care industry is not entitled to secrecy.

The burden of reporting that has arisen in a world burning with conflict and mistrust has cast transparency in its most negative light. Yet I cannot imagine a future health care system in which we do not work in daylight, study openly what we do, and offer patients any windows they want onto the work that affects them. "No secrets" is the new rule in my escape fire.

These are the elements of my escape fire, first draft. I envision a system in which we promise those who depend on us total access to the help they need, in the form they need, when they need it. Our system will promise freedom from the tyranny of individual visits with overburdened professionals as the only way to find a healing relationship; will promise excellence as the standard, valuing such excellence over ill-considered autonomy; will promise safety; and will be capable of nourishing interactions in which information is central, quality is individually defined, control resides with patients, and trust blooms in an open environment.

It is a new system and a lot of the old tools won't work anymore. Those who cling to their old tools and allow our organization to disintegrate will find little sense either in the burning present or in the challenging future. For them, sensemaking will have failed, and the panic of isolation will drive them up a slope that is too far and too steep for them to make it. For the rest, the possibility of invention and the opportunity to make sense—new sense—will open not just routes of escape, but vistas of achievement that the old order could never have imagined.

Further Reading

Cohen, D. K., and Ball, D. L. *Instruction, Capacity and Improvement*. CPRE Research Report no. RR-043. Philadelphia: University of Pennsylvania, Consortium for Policy Research in Education, 1999.

Leape, L. L. "Error in Medicine." *JAMA*, 1994, *272*, 1851–1857.

Maclean, N. *Young Men and Fire*. Chicago: University of Chicago Press, 1992.

Weick, K. E. *Sensemaking in Organizations*. Thousand Oaks, Calif.: Sage, 1995.

9

Dirty Words and Magic Spells

Commentary

Maureen Bisognano

Every now and then, society can be changed by the powerful use of language. Think about the effects of John F. Kennedy's inaugural call to ". . . ask not what your country can do for you; ask what you can do for your country." That sentence crystallized the feelings of a generation, inspiring people to volunteer for the Peace Corps and to commit to a higher level of political and social involvement.

Donald Berwick now offers a linguistic challenge to the status quo in health care. Though he frames the issues in fanciful and funny terms, his message is demanding. Berwick is calling out the need for profound change by focusing on the metaphors we can use for the disorders in our thinking and in our processes.

Let's consider his challenge to the dirty word *discharge*. Although the last decade in health care has focused on mergers and the building of integrated delivery systems in the name of improving patient care, patients are still unnecessarily admitted and discharged within parts of the same integrated system. Waste, delay, and error are built into these handoffs, but most important, how can "discharging" our patients be rationalized in human terms? If medicine is part art and part science, we need to heed

Berwick's call on both terms to eliminate the "discharge process" from health care.

The patient should never feel alone just because she or he is recovering at home or in another care setting. We can build in memory and use the knowledge we gained in our interactions to improve her health. David Gustafson, Professor of Industrial Engineering and Preventive Medicine at the University of Wisconsin, Madison, has built Web-based support systems such as CHESS (Comprehensive Health Enhancement Support System) to keep patients completely integrated with caregivers as they move through different phases and loci of care. The same system has taught clinicians a great deal about the human outcomes of their care of which they were previously unaware and has thus helped to create a vital learning system and improved care.

In addition to building strong continuous feedback loops on the social and human side, we can similarly build them on the scientific side so that physicians and nurses can know how their care turned out in clinical terms. We can learn rapidly, easily, and daily to build more effective care designs when we can link longer-term outcomes with the care we give day to day.

Berwick also asks us to confront the word *compliance*. The word itself invites clinicians to stay rooted in the belief that we prescribe and the patient obeys. Patients do what makes sense to them. If a patient stops taking a hypertensive drug, Berwick invites us to have a conversation with the patient to understand the patient, the environment, and the interactions as a complete system and to avoid judging and labeling because these things are not helpful. The patient might describe intolerable side effects, cost pressures, or scheduling as challenges that drive their decisions. A recent *British Medical Journal* article described the average length of encounters between physicians and patients. The brief nature of these interactions often does not invite the kind of conversations we will need if we are to build true patient partnerships in decision making. We are seeing promising innovations in some clinical practices. Physicians are partnering with nurses and other clinicians to redesign the way care is delivered. E-mail, nurse-led chronic disease clinics, and open access scheduling systems are making care faster and easier for the patients who want to receive care in this way, thereby leaving more time for longer patient interactions for those patients who want and need them.

New designs are needed. Berwick's use of the "dirty words" language is a call to change fundamentally the systems of care and the relationships we build with those we serve. He makes it clear that the problems are large, too large to be named. But so were the social problems to which Kennedy called us. It is my dream that Berwick's words can and will motivate the young people coming into health care careers to see their work in a new way and rise to the challenge of changing the system they have just entered.

Reference

Deveugele, M., Derese, A., van den Brink-Muinen, A., Bensing, J., and DeMaeseneer, J. "Consultation Length in General Practice: Cross-Sectional Study in Six European Countries." *British Medical Journal*, 2002, 325(7362), 472.

Dirty Words and Magic Spells

12th Annual National Forum on Quality Improvement in Health Care

San Francisco, California, December 5, 2000

In the United States, the momentum for change is phenomenal. In our federal government there's great work going on in the Veterans Health Administration, the Bureaus of Primary Care and HIV/AIDS in the Health Resources and Services Administration, and the newly reauthorized Agency for Healthcare Research and Quality. Large systems such as Kaiser, Mayo Clinic, SSM Health Care, Group Health Cooperative of Puget Sound, Premier, VHA, and others are breaking new ground.

And more and more the effort is global.

I want to highlight in particular the amazing work done in the National Health Service in the United Kingdom. Actually, the United Kingdom has given us two great gifts recently. One is the new National Health Service Plan, which offers an inspiring vision of improvement at an immense system level. The other is Harry Potter.

If you want to change health care, you've simply got to read Harry Potter.

For those of you—those two of you—who have escaped the Harry Potter frenzy, let me give you a very brief summary. Harry, who is now twelve, is a wizard, even though he didn't know it until he was eight years old. The world, our world, it turns out, has two types of people in it—magical ones (wizards and witches) and the rest of us, normal ones (muggles). The wizards know there are muggles and live among us, but the muggles don't realize there are wiz-

---

Keynote speech presented at the 12th Annual National Forum on Quality Improvement in Health Care, San Francisco, California, December 5, 2000.

ards, and we muggles go through our pathetic lives thinking that magic is a fantasy.

It isn't. The wizards and witches have their own schools, their own postal system (which consists of owls carrying letters), their own obsession with sports—a sport called Quiddich, which is played on broomsticks and is sort of like lacrosse with no mercy—and their own warfare.

Harry Potter is a good wizard—he's a sort of messiah wizard who thinks he is nothing special even though it's his destiny to save the world. His mentors include the headmaster of Hogwarts, his Wizard School, the kindly Albus Dumbledore, and other elderly, benign wizards who only want to help. Harry's nemesis is Voldemort, a wizard gone bad, sort of a Darth Vader, whose deeds are so terrible that only a few good wizards are even willing to speak his name.

Most people are too scared to refer to him as Voldemort; they call him "he who cannot be named." Voldemort is too bad to name. Voldemort killed Harry Potter's parents, and he is out to get Harry. As of book number four, Voldemort has failed to kill Harry, but the author, J. K. Rowling, promises three more Harry Potter books before she and (who knows?) maybe Harry himself, are finished. Time will tell.

Actually, Harry Potter has two lessons for us in health care. First, he is not afraid to say Voldemort's name; and second, he has magic words to fight Voldemort. Let's take the lessons one at a time.

First, Voldemort's name. Voldemort is exactly the same as health care's quality problems; he's scary to talk about. In fact, most people don't. The problem of quality of care that we need to tackle, the true problem, the true challenge, has a crucial property that we as a nation have not yet faced up to: its size. For most of the people who will determine the future of health care, the problem of quality—the challenge of improvement—is too big to name. And I want to claim that until we name it, we will not solve it.

I actually think we're ready now. Our conviction that we can do better is now strong enough that we can say Voldemort out loud. We can actually describe—clearly and without guilt or fear—the job we intend to tackle.

Of course, not everybody is ready. In fact, in the United States this year many health care leaders have, in my view, actually regressed into a backward-looking battle for old systems, old revenues, and defense of the status quo. I continue to read statements by health care leaders who ought to know better that the last drop of cost has been squeezed out of our bloated system, or that the only way to meet budgets is to cut back on quality. That was nonsense a decade ago and it's nonsense today. We don't need to make that mistake again. We know that the changes we have seen aren't yet close to the changes we need to see.

Reviewing the Basics

Let me describe Voldemort one more time. Some rather prestigious groups have been taking a hard look at the quality of American health care in the past several years and they don't like what they have been finding. An important group is the Institute of Medicine's Roundtable on (IDM's) Health Care Quality, which reported its findings in a landmark lead paper in 1998.[1] Here's what they said:

> Serious and widespread problems exist throughout American medicine. These problems . . . occur in small and large communities alike, in all parts of the country, and with approximately equal frequency in managed care and fee-for-service systems of care. Very large numbers of Americans are harmed as a direct result. Quality of care is the problem, not managed care. Current efforts to improve will not succeed unless we undertake a major, systematic effort to overhaul how we deliver health care services, educate and train clinicians, and assess and improve quality.

These are bold words from a rather conservative organization. The Roundtable classified these pervasive quality problems into three types:

- *Overuse* of procedures and interventions that cannot, on scientific grounds, help the patients who get them—such as 20 percent to 50 percent unnecessary surgery rates for specific procedures, and 30 percent or more overuse of powerful antibiotics

- *Underuse* of treatments and interventions that are known scientifically to be helpful to patients—such as omitting effective vaccines for half of the elderly people in the United States, or failing to use life-extending treatments in half of our heart attack victims

- *Misuse*, which refers to errors in execution of care—mistakes and slip-ups that don't quite fit into the overuse and underuse categories, such as serious medication errors in seven out of every one hundred hospital patients

As you know, the IOM's new Committee on the Quality of Health Care in America published a report on patient safety, *To Err Is Human*, a year ago, which launched a national campaign to improve patient safety, a campaign that's still gathering steam.

The same IOM committee has recently released its full report, *Crossing the Quality Chasm*, which I like to call "the rest of the iceberg." It goes far beyond patient safety, recommending changes to deal with overuse and underuse, as well as addressing issues of service, efficiency, and equity in care.

The report suggests six aims for improving American health care:

- *Safety:* Patients shouldn't suffer injury from the care that is intended to help them. Today thousands of patients are harmed by the care they receive.

- *Effectiveness:* Health care should reliably deliver to patients the care that can, on scientific grounds, help them, and should reliably avoid delivering care that cannot, scientifically, help them. (This amounts to avoiding both underuse and overuse, which according to the Roundtable occur everywhere.)

- *Patient-centeredness:* Health care should be highly individualized. It should meet each and every patient and family respectfully and on their own terms, and the individual's values should guide every decision. (I like the expression, "Every patient is the only patient," which captures this idea.) Today care doesn't respect the individual preferences, needs, and often even the rights of the people it serves.

- *Timeliness:* Health care should respect and not waste the time of either patients or those who provide health care. Care should be responsive. Today it isn't; waiting is everywhere.

- *Efficiency:* Health care should avoid waste, including waste of equipment, supplies, capital, ideas, energy, and other resources that it consumes at the expense of other potential uses. Today we squander a quarter or a third of our health care dollar on scrap, rework, and other defects that help no one.

- *Equity:* Health care should reach all Americans, regardless of their race, ethnicity, wealth, gender, sexual orientation, and place of residence. Today a black baby born in Washington, D.C., has a life expectancy eight years shorter than that of a white baby.

Design Principles: Knowledge-Based, Patient-Centered, Systems-Minded

The IOM says that these problems are neither acceptable nor inevitable. But the IOM also concludes that the American health care system, as currently designed, can't possibly achieve substantial improvements in these six dimensions. We can have substantially better care, but we can't get *there* from *here*. The problem is design. The system we have lacks three basic properties that are preconditions to effective, continual improvements.

First, we need our care to be *knowledge-based*. Today it isn't. The gap between scientific knowledge and actual practice is very wide.

Second, we need our care to be *fully centered on patients*—putting patients firmly in control. Today's care isn't patient-centered. It is designed for acute illnesses, not for the chronic diseases that are now our mainstream morbidities. It places patients in a helpless, dependent posture instead of encouraging self-efficacy and assertiveness.

Third, we need care to be *systems-minded*, always connected, flowing gently and seamlessly without delays, obstructions, or failures of coordination. Today's care is not. Instead of flow we have waits and delays everywhere. We forget crucial information and values as our patients and their loved ones try to negotiate their way from one high-tech island to another.

If we got that right—making our care knowledge-based, patient-centered, and systems-minded—the rest would follow much more easily; our progress toward the six improvement aims would be far better and faster. But we don't have it right.

The experiences that my wife and I have had in the course of her recent serious illness have made us acutely aware of the dependency, fear, and uncertainty we felt as a patient and family in a system that too often let us down.

Instead of knowledge-based care centered on excellence, we found enormous variation and inconsistency, and obvious failures on the part of the good people who gave us care to learn from their own collective, accumulated experience and ours.

Instead of patient-centered care, we found ourselves enmeshed in onerous rules and assaults on our dignity, and we found our caregivers too often more interested in explaining how something must be done instead of asking us how we needed it to be done. We felt forgotten.

Instead of a smoothly flowing and constantly coordinated system—instead of a system at all—we found that we were sailing from medical island to medical island, carrying incomplete messages to institutions and people who never seemed to understand that they were part of a whole, and that we depended, literally for our lives, on the whole even more than on the parts.

And we are not alone. Many others have shared with me their equally discouraging stories.

For example, an experienced health care executive wrote:

> My wife's mother . . . had six admissions last year and spent over sixty days of the final year of her life as an inpatient. We were afraid, confused, and often angry about the many systemic breakdowns. . . . The enormity of the problems was truly driven home for me when a new physician on her case indicated one-by-one a number of treatment options for my mother-in-law. Every one was rejected after we indicated to the doctor that all of his approaches had been tried previously with no positive result and often adverse consequences. He finally offered, "Maybe I should read the chart"!!! The health care team had little collective wisdom. . . . I am becoming increasingly convinced that we have a health care industry leadership problem that is so big it is almost impossible to get your arms around it.

Just a month ago, one of the most distinguished professors of medicine in America pulled me aside to tell me that his wife had been hospitalized in a great university hospital. He said he was frightened to leave her bedside and decided not to. He said, "I just felt that if I was not there, something awful would happen to her. I needed to defend her from the care." I have heard the same from dozens and dozens of health care professionals.

This is chilling. It is even more chilling because the professor was right to stand guard for his wife. I know how dedicated our doctors, nurses, technicians, pharmacists, respiratory therapists, managers, and executives are. They are wonderful. They are us. Yet I hear a voice of alarm from the people we would help—including us when we need help too—that tells me in poetic form what I already knew numerically: the care is wrong. Too often, in too many places, while hurting too many people, the care is not pretty good; it is not even fair. It is wrong. *That* is our Voldemort.

In a recent article comparing quality of care in teaching hospitals with quality of care in nonteaching hospitals, the investigators studied more than two hundred thousand Medicare patients with acute myocardial infarctions.[2] They selected those who were "ideal candidates" for four life-extending treatments: reperfusion at admission, aspirin during their hospitalizations, and beta-blockers and ACE inhibitors at discharge.

What they found and reported was an advantage in quality of care in teaching hospitals. Look at the beta-blocker story. Indeed, patients in teaching hospitals fared better. Among them, 49 percent of ideal candidates for beta-blockers got them, compared with 36 percent in nonteaching hospitals. The authors' conclusion: quality of care is better in teaching hospitals.

Yes, but wait a minute. Is that the right headline? How about, "Defect rate over 50 percent in even the best of our hospitals?"

Voldemort looks like this: today in the United States of America, average citizens, even those with health care coverage and access, cannot count on receiving high-quality health care. Most, if they are sick enough for long enough, will experience and suffer from poor quality—not just errors, but poor quality. Let me say it again: the average American does not reliably receive care of high quality.

And by and large, with the sole and welcome exception of recent concerns about safety, the scale of the quality problem remains ignored—unnamed. Except here, now.

Mark Twain commented on Richard Wagner's music this way: "It is not as bad as it sounds." Our nation—with forty million uninsured; with vast levels of unnecessary care; with yawning gaps in the provision of basic, effective forms of care; with waits and delays everywhere; with a public frustrated by unresponsiveness; and with costs 30 percent above those of any other nation on Earth—continues to seem to believe that our health care quality is not as bad as we absolutely know it to be. It *is* as bad as it sounds.

Now this presents us with an enormous dilemma. In fact, naming the problem is necessary, but it can leave you feeling pretty bad if you stop there. We have therefore got two problems, not one: the first is to face reality, the second is to preserve hope.

There is some hope. For example, compare the study of MI care noted earlier with that same study design replicated in the eight hospitals of the Veterans Health Administration Heartland Network.[3] Many of us feel that the Veterans Administration is setting the pace in the nation for demonstrating a real, systemic focus on quality as a priority, and results like these are the reason. In these eight hospitals, average beta-blocker use reached 96 percent, and the worst hospital of the eight was still over 90 percent. How did they do that? And could we all do it too?

How can we possibly name, without guilt but with clarity, courage, and direction, the central point that the health care system has to change, not a little but a lot? How can we possibly face reality and be hopeful at the same time? Harry Potter is no fool. He is willing to face down Voldemort because he has a plan. Magic words. So can we.

Magic Words

Let me tell you where I'm going with this. Harry Potter knows, because Dumbledore told him, that the magic words are woven together with thoughts. They work because of what Harry believes, not just because of what he says. If you ever took Psych 101, you know that we all use magic words. Our words encode our beliefs and make them seem to be facts. We say what we believe, and then we believe what we say.

And to beat Voldemort, what we believe today won't be strong enough. The old thoughts don't do it; the old words, encoding the old thoughts, cast the wrong spell. I want to question some words, the ones we have created to maintain the thoughts that won't do any longer. The changes we need to make are vast, because Voldemort is so strong. We can name him safely, but only if we learn to think, and therefore to speak, differently.

Now, once you get that idea—that improving health care is going to require ways of thinking so different from the ways we use now that they will require our very words to change—you will be on your way to new vocabularies—magic words—far better than those I may choose. But let me give you a start, by way of example. I'll tell you a few of the words—six words—that I don't think work anymore—dirty words that cast bad spells—and I'll show you some new ones, with new spells, better spells. Welcome to Hogwarts.

DIRTY WORD 1: *Discharge*

The word *discharge* in health care might as well be about sewage discharge. We are sending it away. We are done with it. Good riddance. In health care, the idea of discharge isn't compatible with our being knowledge based, patient centered, or systems minded. The patients' journeys do not end for them in any important respect when they exit our buildings. The problem too big to name is that we pretend this isn't so; we pretend that it is all right to organize our care around the needs of the care system instead of around the needs of the patient.

Health care has forgotten to ask about the long haul. It's as if we don't want to know. Those who suffer are "admitted" and then "discharged" by a system whose scissors cut paths across continuous existence. The idea of discharge poisons systems thinking, prevents us from centering on patients, and keeps us from gaining knowledge of how well we are doing.

Discharge (and even *admit*) are dirty words. Voldemort's words. They reflect our commitment to discontinuity. They create a commitment to discontinuity, discontinuity too big to name. What's missing is memory.

When my children were born I did not "admit" them, and I intend not to "discharge" them, even though they will make their own way in the world. If I don't admit or discharge my children, what do I do that marks transitions? I remember them when they leave me for a time. I greet them when they return. I call them often, and they call me. And when we are apart we think of one another. If the dirty word is *discharge*, maybe the magic words are *greet* and *remember*. Today, we can easily awe our patients, but we have trouble greeting them. We remember their insurance numbers but forget their names.

What if we didn't write discharge notes but kept albums? For our most vulnerable patients, those with the greatest fear or whose suffering will not end, what if we called from time to time just to see how they are doing? Let's find a word that means, "Even though you are leaving my building or my office, I know I am part of your life now. I remember you. In any way that proves useful for me to enter your life again, I will do that—upon your request and without hesitation." The dirty word is *discharge*; the magic word, *remember*.

DIRTY WORD 2: *Compliance*

Compliance is the property of a material that allows it to bend around other materials, to change its shape. Bubble gum and silly putty are really compliant. Steel isn't. Nor is an oak beam. The thesaurus says that synonyms of *compliant* are *obedient, submissive,* and *yielding*.

Do we want patients of steel or of bubble gum? Which do you like? "Mrs. Mary Jones has diabetes, and when it comes to her treatment she is obedient and submissive." Or "Mrs. Mary Jones has diabetes, and when it comes to her treatment she has a mind of her own; she takes charge; she asserts herself."

Noncompliance does not signal that the patient has a problem. It signals that we who wish to help them have a problem. It means that we are missing some boat—that we do not understand. Maybe the problem too big to name—hidden by the dirty word *compliance*—is that we get to do our work in ignorance of the true needs of the patient. It is that we get paid whether or not we have helped. We get at some point to shift the blame for failure, even when the failure is ours—not to have heard, not to have learned, not to have complied—when *we* have not complied with the astounding and beautiful variety that our patients bring to us. The compliance we should aspire to is ours with the patient, not the patient's with us.

In a true alliance with the patients we serve there isn't any room for the spells that the word *compliance* casts. The spells deny us knowledge of the patient as an individual, convert the quest for patient-centeredness into a distancing struggle for control, and fragment our teamwork with our patients. They create fragmentation too big to name.

Compliance is a dirty word; the magic word is *choice* or *agreement*. The word we need would cast a spell of reliability and robustness, and unstinting respect for the patient. Not, "Mr. Smith did not comply with the prescription," but rather, "Mr. Smith disagreed with the prescription." Not, "I prescribed the medication, but Mr. Smith did not follow the instructions," but, "Mr. Smith chose not to take it because he knew better."

DIRTY WORD 3: *You can't manage it if you can't measure it.*

Dirty Word 3 is actually a dirty phrase, not a word.

I tried it out on my daughter Jessica. Since I want to manage my relationship with her well, I decided to create a balanced scorecard and collect data systematically. We carefully defined the data elements, six key indicators: minutes together per week; voice tone and level (her voice tone plus my voice tone, divided by two); transportation adequacy; telephone costs; arguments related to nutrition and substance use; and hugs, adjusted for squeeze tone and length. Last week I got a 63, but I don't agree with the severity adjustment. I had a tough week at work.

This is stupid. Jessica wouldn't stand for it, and I wouldn't do it. Yet I care deeply about my quality as a parent, seek always to improve, and I would go so far as to say that I manage my parenting all the time—if, that is, *managing* is the opposite of *neglecting*.

Dr. Paul Batalden of Dartmouth Medical School has pointed out that when we talk about managing something, that something is, we mean to say, a reality. A real-world thing. "Parenting" Jessica is close to the name of the real-world thing I mean to manage, but it is actually more than that. It is nameless. It involves love, and relationship, and fun, and safety, and companionship. We can give it a name, *parenting*, for convenience, but the name isn't the thing. It's a shadow of the thing.

Friedrich Nietzsche said, "That for which we find words is something already dead in our hearts. There is always a kind of contempt in the act of speaking." Edward de Bono has written, "Language is the graveyard of concepts." We love or care about a reality that is beyond naming, far too complex. Our name, though we need it, kills the reality by putting it into a box. This is convenient, but it is wrong.

It is the same with health care. Imagine that someone you love has newly diagnosed breast cancer. What does she need? Don't name what she needs. Imagine it. *Image* it. It can't be said in a word. It would be a story, a long story. Probably a lifelong story. The story would be about fear and safety, about pain and comfort, about self-image and self-esteem and embarrassment and secrecy. It would be about drugs and radiation and surgery, but also about having her hand held and about holding her children. What she needs may just barely be "storyable," but it is not conceivably namable. When we name it, we kill it.

But we cannot live in the world with stories only. We don't have enough time. We condense stories and we save time with codes—our words and labels are the codes.

What does a woman with newly diagnosed breast cancer need? Quickly! I don't have time to hear the whole story, and besides, it would make me uncomfortable to know all about her suffering.

So we say she needs "disease management." She needs "evidence-based medicine." She needs "best practices."

It is dead. The story is dead. These words are very pale, very one-dimensional ghosts of a reality with infinite important dimensions. Maybe we can use art to try to stay in touch with the reality. T. S. Eliot said, "Poetry communicates before it is understood." Labels certainly don't do the job.

But even the labels are too complicated. We seem to want not just to *summarize* reality in words, but to *manage* it, so we have to hammer the words into a more concrete form—something we can get our hands on, not just labels. So we measure.

Suffering becomes *illness* when it crosses over into language, and *illness* in language becomes *temperature* when it crosses over into measurement. The relief of suffering becomes *satisfaction* or *functional status* in language. Satisfaction becomes a questionnaire in measurement, and function becomes an SF-36 Health Survey. My wife, Ann, becomes a myelitis case, and her myelitis care becomes a length of stay. And her SF-36 score is 26. My wife becomes a score of 26. Says who? Inexperienced young doctors manage the patients' numbers; wise old ones ask the patient how things are going.

At its best, measurement can give us a vague, shadowy outline of what we care about. At its worst, it disconnects us from the meaning entirely. Always remember: the word is not the story, and the measurement is not even so much as the word. To paraphrase Nietzsche: There is always a kind of contempt in the act of measuring. We err badly, we do harm, when we confuse the measurement with the reality. It is two giant steps removed. It is two universes removed. A number is as far from a story as a wedding ring is from a marriage.

Of course we need measuring to help us in our journeys. But it can't help if we forget the stories. I don't believe that we cannot manage what we cannot measure. I believe that we cannot improve when we cannot tell a story.

There is a deep and costly confusion about this in our evolving health care industry. The current stories are indeed wrong, but the secret to the new stories does not lie in measuring. It lies in remembering. The problem too big to name is that the stories are real, and powerful, and deeply painful. If we named it, we might even have to begin to wonder if medicine itself ought to be the preeminent discipline in a patient-centered health system. We are here together to do a very, very difficult job. How nice it would be—how comfortable—if it were indeed just about the numbers.

I have a favorite quotation from a speech by Robert Kennedy in the 1960s. It is about another measurement, the gross national product (GNP):

> Our gross national product is now over eight hundred billion dollars a year. But that GNP—if we should judge America by it—counts air pollution and cigarette advertising, and ambulances to clear our highways of carnage. It counts special locks for our doors and the jails for those who break them. It counts the destruction of our redwoods and the loss of our natural wonder in chaotic sprawl. It counts napalm and the cost of a nuclear warhead, and armored cars for police who fight riots in our streets. It counts Whitman's rifle and Speck's knife, and the television programs which glorify violence in order to sell toys to our children.
>
> Yet the gross national product does not allow for the health of our children, the quality of their education, or the joy of their play. It does not include the beauty of our poetry or the strength of our marriages; the intelligence of our public debate or the integrity of our public officials.

It measures neither our wit nor our courage; neither our
wisdom nor our learning; neither our compassion nor
our devotion to our country; it measures everything, in
short, except that which makes life worthwhile.[4]

You cannot manage it if you cannot measure it? Nonsense. Nonsense at least until we remember the stories. Which leads me to
Dirty Word 4.

DIRTY WORD 4: *Accountability*

The confusion of measurement with reality is first cousin to
another confusion: confusing *counting* with *relationship*. *Accountability* is Voldemort's word. If we rely on accountability as the key
to improvements in health care, we will fail. The problem—the glo-
rious problem—is that people, in the end, decide what they will do.
There is no such thing as managing another person's behavior. It is
a nonsense expression.

We want patient safety in America, so the debate rages as to
how we could hold people and organizations accountable for safety
levels so their behavior will change. I have seen three superb, inspiring examples of a focus on safety as a passionate and effective concern; each has used accountability as a tool, but none has depended
on accountability for its energy, for its ultimate effect.

The first example is the one set by Paul O'Neill, Chairman of
Alcoa, which last year became, statistically, the safest company in
the world, from the viewpoint of worker injuries.[5] You can see
Alcoa's injury rate if you want to by logging onto the Web; they
voluntarily put it there for all to see. When O'Neill took over
Alcoa more than fifteen years ago, he learned on almost his first
day on the job that a twenty-one-year-old boy had been killed the
day before in an Alcoa plant by a spring-loaded armature that struck
his head. The next day O'Neill faced his own senior staff and
announced, "We killed a boy yesterday, and we will not do it again."

Every day since, O'Neill has personally reviewed the prior day's injuries at Alcoa.

The second example is from Bill Rupp, CEO of Luther Midelfort Clinic, a division of Mayo Clinic in Eau Claire, Wisconsin. While others have debated the malpractice issues associated with errors with the mandatory or voluntary reporting of errors, and with how exactly to define an error, Bill has for three years now driven his organization day by day to identify and prevent patient injuries. He started this effort before the IOM hype, and he will continue it long after the headlines have gone away.

The third example I saw just two months ago on a visit to Japan. I was speaking at a conference on patient safety there, where there is a dawning awakening that quality management in health care would be a good idea. The closing speaker was Dr. Matabee Maeda, chairman of the Maeda Construction Company, a two-time Deming Prize winner in Japan. Dr. Maeda is a dignified, highly respected Japanese industrial leader, and he's currently president of the Japanese Society for Quality Control. He had listened patiently for a whole day to Japanese health care leaders considering whether they should tackle patient safety as an issue, what the risks of lawsuits might be, and whether it would be financially wise. It sounded a lot like the United States.

Then Dr. Maeda spoke, and he described his own commitment to worker safety in his company. He recalled the critical event that had focused his attention—a tunnel construction accident in 1976 in which thirty-six workers died. As he spoke, twenty-five years after that tragedy, standing in front of a health care audience of four hundred people he did not know, Dr. Maeda began to weep. "You see," he said, "the memory still brings tears to me." He said, "Please, make your patients safe."

The tears matter. Probably many of you, most of you, will think me naive. You will say that I overinvest my hopes in intrinsic human motives. I respectfully disagree. I will bet every time on Dr. Maeda's tears over anyone's public reporting system. Transparency and the appearance of accountability may be a helpful, even a necessary, precondition to the change we want. Paul O'Neill gets daily reports on injuries in Alcoa, and everybody knows it. Yet I promise you, reporting by itself is far, far from sufficient.

Emotional sterility will doom the patient safety movement. Tears will nourish it. Voldemort's view of accountability amputates people from their own tears. They become afraid, not that patients will die, but rather that the numbers will hurt them.

We will be truly safer, and we will improve our care, when health care executives, chiefs of medicine, head nurses—when all of us—connect our actions to what we feel when we realize that our patients are confused, that their pain is unrelieved, that they die sooner than they need to.

The Institute for Healthcare Improvement organized a Breakthrough Series project last year on improving care at the end of life. I remember one baseline report from a participating hospital that measured the time between arrival and the first dose of pain medication for terminally ill patients admitted to that hospital for the purpose of pain relief. The median delay was 110 minutes. The number haunts me. Have you ever been in severe pain? Pain that you feared would not go away? Can you imagine lying on a gurney in an emergency room in pain, as an "expected admission," there for relief of your pain, and having 110 minutes tick by before your first dose of medicine? Sometime instead of a speech I think I will just tell that story, and then sit quietly with my audience for 110 minutes, waiting.

Don't misunderstand me. I agree that it can be helpful if there are consequences for our actions—accountability. But my plea is that that is not at all sufficient. As measurement can pluck the heart from a story, accountability can pluck the soul from our intentions. The leader who thinks it is enough to create report cards and contingent rewards misses the biggest and hardest opportunity of leadership itself—to help people discover and celebrate the meaning in their work. Voldemort thinks that the magic is in the accounting. We know that the magic is in the meaning.

DIRTY WORD 5: *No margin, no mission*

And so comes Dirty Word 5, also a phrase. It sounds so realistic and hard-headed. I warn you: wrong spell, black magic, Voldemort loves it. It marks a problem too big to name. So, think again.

I have been thinking for some time about the best way to state our purpose in medicine in its highest form. The best I can come up with is this: *relieve suffering*. This includes prevention, because I mean by this not just the suffering that is, but the suffering that will be if we don't act to prevent it. True north is to relieve suffering among those who come to us, or could come to us, for help.

Now, let's take this idea—relieve suffering—and play it back through Dirty Word 5: "No margin, no relief of suffering." It doesn't sound quite right, because it isn't right. It is as if the people who make cookies said, "No margin, no cookies." Or an airline said, "No margin, no flying."

That sounds a little silly. Wouldn't you want to tell the airline, "You have it backwards. It's, 'No flying, no margin'"? Margin, the surrogate idea for corporate vitality—the securing of a future—comes from doing your job right for people who want you to do that job and are willing to pay you to do it. I think we need to see margin as a consequence of the pursuit of purpose. We need to *make* margin the consequence of the pursuit of purpose.

This is much more than rhetoric. It is both the basic guiding moral framework and the heartwood business strategy of the modern quality movement. Many industries and many more companies have gotten into deep trouble by checking their margins before their purposes, instead of seeking margins by improving their pursuit of purpose.

If our purpose is to relieve suffering, then I say, "No relief, no margin." Actually, I say, "No relief, good riddance."

The problem too big to name is that the system is set up backwards right now. Suppose a patient with congestive heart failure escapes effective treatment and ends up in the hospital. Under most current payment systems, as the suffering increases, so does the mar-

gin. The system of care gets paid—makes a profit—because of its
own fragmentation and defects—its failures to employ knowledge-
based, patient-centered, systems-minded care. It is not just not paid
to do well; it is rewarded for doing poorly. This is an exceedingly
uncomfortable reality, exceedingly hard to name. We continue to
build, support, and encourage low-volume, high-tech care programs
even though we know with near certainty that outcomes will
worsen as a result.

By the way, if you really care about the money, the biggest
opportunity for margin and survival in American health care is the
tough and disciplined examination of our own activities through
the lens of health care's mission. If we could all together develop the
force and clarity to ask of each and every step we take—every building we build, every machine we plug in, every program we start or
end, every drug, every rule, every hour of training, every minute of
work, every message we send, and every target we set—the simple
question, "Will this further relieve the suffering?" then I believe we
would stand the greatest possible chance of getting this sick system
back on its feet.

By this measure, the waste is phenomenal, simply phenomenal.
Drugs, tests, and surgery that cannot help. Forms and records that
no one uses and that add complexity beyond repair. Idle capital and
downtime, even while we expand low-volume facilities with predictably poorer outcomes. Redundant inspections and reviews.
Processes with twenty steps that could be cut down to three. The
constant rework and burden of tracking down missing information,
missing people, and missing supplies.

I stand by my estimate that if we were to use relief of suffering
as the primary index of value, 30 to 40 percent of American health
care expenses are pure waste—$300 billion to $400 billion at a minimum. At least this proportion of our expenditures relieves no suffering at all, and much of it adds to suffering. The recovery of waste
through a focus on purpose is, by an order of magnitude, the largest
opportunity for financial gain in the American health care system,

whether we choose to return that gain to taxpayers or investors, to reinvest it in even better health care, or to use it to build better public schools.

The problem too big to name is that the American health care system and those who pay for it have lost their focus on the relief of suffering as its primary reason for existence and its primary strategy for survival. "No margin, no mission" won't work; wrong spell. I think we have to explore what it means to say instead, "No mission, no margin."

DIRTY WORD 6: *Taseki*

Dirty Word 6 is Japanese. I learned it from my Japanese friend and colleague Dr. Naruo Uehara, who hosted me on my recent trip to his country. I don't know a single synonym in English, but *taseki*, if I get it right, means, "The dog ate my homework." "I didn't do it." "Not my problem." Or maybe, "Somebody ought to do something about this." "*Your* burden," it means, "not mine." *Taseki*.

It is the standard defensive posture for inaction on the quality frontier. *Taseki* is the long list of reasons why we cannot openly address patient safety—the malpractice lawyers, the inevitability of hazards, the problems of measurement, or the resistance of "those doctors." It is behind the claim that our outrageous health care costs come from insatiable American appetites for care, that doctors won't "buy in" to change, that we could make changes if only there were no unions, or improve profits if only the payers would pay us more. It blames our inaction on the Joint Commission yesterday, on the Balanced Budget Act today, and on unwise consumers tomorrow. It resists authentic inquiry about how the health care systems of Canada, Holland, Norway, Sweden, and a dozen other Western nations do so well with so much less expense by saying, "We are different, case closed."

The opposite of *taseki* in Japanese is *jiseki*. "My burden." "I'll handle it." "I can, I will." It's *The Little Engine That Could* for children, Dunkirk or Normandy or Americans on the moon for adults.

The shouldering of responsibility—*jiseki*—is part of the train-ing and romance of the health care professions at their best. Alan Gregg, for decades the head of health care programs at the Rock-efeller Foundation, wrote: "Sometimes it helps if you remind the desperately ill patient that it is the doctor's job to do the worry-ing, because the patient is too busy being sick to take on anything additional."

When was the last time America's health care leaders reminded the public we serve that it need not worry about our caring? That we will do the worrying? That we know they are too busy suffering—being sick, at risk, or frightened—to take on anything additional? Joanne Lynn of Americans for Better Care of the Dying calls this "making promises," and it is *jiseki*, taking the burden, not *taseki*, passing the buck. What promises have we made?

Jiseki makes mincemeat of some other words that *taseki* likes. If we bear the burden, we cannot think much of claims that patients expect too much, or that our system would perform better if con-sumers took more risks. If we wanted to talk about "partnering" with patients, we would have to mean it, not use it as code for blaming them for their choices. We would bear the burden of explaining our work, of resolving confusion, and of revealing our errors. We would seek excellence, not excuses. We would figure out how to use bet-ter the abundant resources we have instead of complaining about the resources we lack. We would be optimists, not victims. We would talk far less about payment for old things and far more about revenues for new ones; far less about costs and far more about waste. We would tell our publics not how bad things are, but how good we will make them. We would make far fewer explanations, and far more promises.

Quality is *jiseki*, our burden. Our care will improve when and if we decide it will improve, not before, and not without us. We got to the moon because we decided to; we did not decide to because we knew how. We will improve health care only as much as we *decide* to improve—not a particle more.

I think soon, if not now, our nation may have had its fill of excuses about health care. We hold in trust nearly $1.5 trillion a year, put in our hands for the sole and worthy purpose of relieving the suffering of our fellow human beings. In giving us that resource, and in trusting us enough to hope that we will use it wisely, the public we serve has done its job, completely. They are too busy needing us to take on anything additional. The job of meeting that need is now our burden, *jiseki*, up to us, or we ought to give them back the money, with our apology that we, not they, have failed.

Look. I know my message is tough, and in some sense I want to apologize. The problem is the reality. The reality is not good, not anywhere good enough. I just don't think we are going to have the will to make the changes we need unless we face that reality squarely, and give it a name. It's Voldemort. It's intimidating.

But hope matters too. We *are* ready. And what can bridge us from the reality to hope is clear: it is change. It's deep change—change in what we do and change in what we think. But it is all possible. It requires only that we think again. Our words are not our masters. We are boss, not them. We made them, and we can change them. Not *discharge*, but *remember*. Not *compliant* patients, but strong ones, oak beam patients, taking control, trusting themselves. Measurement is crucial, of course, but please remember that measurement involves a kind of contempt. Our measurements will mislead us if we forget the stories. I guess we need accountability, but not at the expense of our deeper, more reliable motivations. If you see, "No margin, no mission," strike it out and put "Mission, period." Or equally good, "Relieve suffering . . . improve function . . . to survive." And if someone says their dog ate their homework, teach them *jiseki*, because you don't get any credit from me at all for *taseki*. Sorry.

Of course, if you want extra credit at Hogwarts, don't use my new words, use yours. The harder your new words are for me to understand at first, the better I'll like it. I especially love new jargon; it makes me think. And every so often I find in a new word a new spell, one that reminds me that just when I thought I knew all the possibilities, another one appears like magic, within reach.

Just don't be scared. I'm not. I'm not scared of Voldemort. I'm willing to speak his name: Voldemort, Voldemort, Voldemort. See . . . I'm still here. He's out there. Go get him!

Notes

1. Chassin, M. R., and Galvin, R. W. "The Urgent Need to Improve Health Care Quality: Institute of Medicine National Roundtable on Health Care Quality." JAMA, 1998, 280(11), 1000–1005.

2. Allison, J. J., Kiefe, C. I., Weissman, N. W., and others. "Relationship of Hospital Teaching Status with Quality of Care and Mortality for Medicare Patients with Acute Myocardial Infarction." JAMA, 2000, 284(10), 1256–1262.

3. Vincent Alvarez, MD, Medical Director, Veterans Health Administration Heartland Network, personal communication, October 2000.

4. Kennedy, R. F. RFK: Collected Speeches. New York: Viking, 1993.

5. Workplace Safety at Alcoa. Business Case no. 9–692–042. Cambridge, Mass.: Harvard Business School, 1991.

Further Reading

Bloom, H. Shakespeare: The Invention of the Human. New York: Riverhead Books, 1998.

de Bono, E. Lateral Thinking: Creativity Step by Step. New York: Harper & Row, 1970.

Gregg, A. For Future Doctors. Chicago: University of Chicago Press, 1957.

Institute of Medicine. To Err Is Human: Building a Safer Health System. Washington, D.C.: National Academies Press, 1999.

Institute of Medicine. Crossing the Quality Chasm: A New Health System for the Twenty-First Century. Washington, D.C.: National Academies Press, 2001.

Rowling, J. K. Harry Potter and the Sorcerer's Stone. (Book 1). New York: Scholastic, 1998.

10

· ·

Every Single One

Commentary

Howard Hiatt

This eloquent and moving address takes us from a project to cure patients with multi-drug-resistant tuberculosis (MDR-TB) in a barrio in Lima, Peru, to programs designed to achieve perfection in health care systems in the United States and in other industrialized countries, and back to Peru. Both objectives seemed (and seem) to many "experts" unattainable. In both situations, Berwick tells us, a prerequisite to success is ensuring that every patient in every setting is treated as though he or she is the only one.

Contrary to the predictions of many specialists around the world, the first goal has already been realized. Impoverished patients with MDR-TB have been treated in a project organized and directed by Partners in Health, a nonprofit Boston-based group directed by Drs. Jim Kim and Paul Farmer, and its Lima partner, *Socios en Salud*, led by Dr. Jaime Bayona. The project has cured more than 80 percent of its patients. In so doing, its leaders have brought a skeptical World Health Organization to embrace their approach. One key element in their success, Berwick tells us, is the total commitment of Dr. Bayona, who directs the program, to every single one of his patients—hence the title of this talk.

The second goal, perfection in health care, is what Berwick expects will emerge in a project overseen by his Institute for

Healthcare Improvement (IHI). With the support of The Robert Wood Johnson Foundation, the movement of the system of health care toward perfection has begun, Berwick says, in several sites in the United States and abroad, guided by principles set forth in a recent report from the Institute of Medicine, *Crossing the Quality Chasm: A New Health System for the Twenty-First Century*. That report presents six attributes essential for improvement: safety, effectiveness, patient-centeredness, timeliness, efficiency, and equity. But unswerving attention to every single patient in every single site will also be critical to success, Berwick maintains, as critical as it has been to the cure of drug-resistant tuberculosis.

Berwick is of course aware that many involved in the delivery of medical services (and even more involved in receiving them) doubt that perfection can be achieved. In his inimitable style, he interviews one (hypothetical) skeptical medical colleague, as well as one who has signed on. He respectfully deals with the first, although he is unable to bring him around. Even we converts, how-ever, are left with the suspicion that achieving perfection in the health care system will be more difficult than curing MDR-TB. Nevertheless, those of us who have followed Berwick's activities carefully over the past decade are strongly tempted to wager that as Berwick's approaches are implemented, perfect systems of health care will emerge.

The IHI approach to problems in our health care system is first to describe and measure them, then to identify methods for dealing with them, next to test and modify those methods, and after improvements are achieved, to disseminate them. Berwick and IHI are already involved in applying their formula of hard work, smart strategies, persistence, courage, and continuing assessment to the control of MDR-TB in Peru. Early results suggest that IHI approaches that lead to reduction of mortality rates after coronary artery bypass surgery or of waiting time in doctors' offices are also effective in disseminating effective MDR-TB treatment programs in a Third World country. Although the experiment is thus far lim-ited to Lima and a few outlying areas of Peru, there are compelling reasons to believe that it will work for disseminating such programs around the world. Further, what works for MDR-TB, Berwick believes, will work equally well for HIV treatment programs and other health scourges.

Those who know Berwick well will recognize that he uses this address to promote his deeply held belief that health care is a right of every individual everywhere. His conviction derives from his respect for every human being, whatever her station, wherever his home. Berwick has long expressed his aspiration to direct a large part of his work to the health needs of the poorest people, wherever they may be. This address is an announcement that that phase of his career is under way.

Berwick begins and ends this address with stirring references to the 9/11 catastrophe—and appropriately so, for a commitment to the delivery of health care of quality for all citizens of the world seems potentially a far more appropriate and effective response to the widespread suspicions about our nation than many of the initiatives that have been suggested by others.

Every Single One

13th Annual National Forum on Quality Improvement in Health Care

Orlando, Florida, December 11, 2001

Lima, Peru, is a sprawling city of eight million people. It sits in a bowl, like Los Angeles, on the Pacific seacoast. North, east, and south of the ocean, the city is slowly climbing the dry hillsides, where its poorest people raise shacks to live in: first cardboard; then, over time, wood and stone; and if they do well, eventually concrete.

Carabayllo is one of the poorest of these shantytowns, on the slopes to the northeast of Lima, with one hundred thousand people. Ten years ago, a Jesuit priest, Father Jack Roussin, came to Carabayllo and decided to make building the community there his life's work.

In 1994, two young doctors from Harvard Medical School, Jim Yong Kim and Paul Farmer, who knew Father Jack, came to Peru to help him. Jim and Paul are heroes of mine, and I want to take a few minutes to tell you about them.

Jim and Paul are both anthropologists and infectious disease physicians. Almost two decades ago, when they were still medical students, they decided to spend part of their lives to help the world's poorest people. They job-shared in residency, and now, Harvard faculty, they give half their time to the normal work of American

---

Keynote speech presented at the 13th Annual National Forum on Quality Improvement in Health Care, Orlando, Florida, December 11, 2001.

This talk was given on December 11, 2001, three months to the hour after the terrorist attacks in New York, Virginia, and Pennsylvania. I began by suggesting to the audience that we stand for a moment to reflect together. I then acknowledged the special effort and commitment those present had made by attending the IHI National Forum at a time when travel was tough. If the people they serve understood why these dedicated health care workers came, those people would have thanked them too.

academic medicine and the other half to building programs and infrastructure in some of the least developed parts of the world. In 1993, the MacArthur Foundation gave Paul Farmer one of its so-called "genius awards," and he donated the money to an organization that he and Jim had started six years earlier, called Partners in Health.

Today, Partners in Health has more than 350 people working with it in health-promoting activities in Haiti, Russia, inner city Boston, Mexico, and Peru. It's attracting a lot of young people. One out of every five Harvard Medical School students is involved somewhere with Partners' work. My own oldest daughter, Jessica, spent last summer, the summer of her freshman year in college, in Carabayllo, working for Partners.

Paul and Jim are very much in tune with the theme of this year's National Forum—"We, the people. . . ." What Jim and Paul think, and what gives Partners in Health its mission, is that the poorest people in the world have a right to health care that's as good as the health care you people in this room get. Paul and Jim's real goal is social justice—equity in the world. But they wanted to start somewhere, so they started with health care.

They picked an especially tough issue within health care to push their theory—the problem of multi-drug-resistant tuberculosis, or MDR-TB. The tuberculosis germ is inside the bodies of one-third of the people in the world—almost all of them poor. The world has one new TB case per second . . . eight million a year. TB joins AIDS and malaria as one of the largest infectious scourges on the planet; it will kill two million people this year, thirty-five million between now and the year 2020.

One out of every twenty people infected with tuberculosis now has a form of the disease that poses a gigantic threat. If it ever broke out, even in our country, it could cause a pandemic. Multi-drug-resistant tuberculosis, just as it sounds, is a tuberculosis germ that has learned resistance, through mutation, to the drugs that cure regular, nonresistant TB. You can treat MDR-TB, but that requires a symphony of drugs, used together in overlapping attacks on the resistant germ. If you're lucky, and if you get the right combination of drugs, taken without fail, with the right management of their inevitable side effects, your MDR-TB can be cured. If you get the wrong drugs, only the usual drugs, or no drugs, odds are you'll waste away and be dead in a year or two.

You are lucky. If you happen to get MDR-TB, you will probably get cured. You would have to try pretty hard right now to get it, of course. You could do it on the right airplane trip or on the right National Geographic tour or on the right Peace Corps mission or if you have business in Moscow and the man across the aisle from you on the subway car has recently been released from prison. Here is what would happen to you. You would get a fever, perhaps start coughing. You'd tell your doctor about your travel history, get a chest X-ray and a skin test, and then fail your usual pneumonia treatment. So your doctor would get a sputum sample from you, and find TB. You would not respond well to the initial course of antituberculosis medications, so your doctor would refer you for a consult with an infectious disease specialist, who would study the antibiotic sensitivity patterns of your sputum culture. Then just the right combination of medicines would be prescribed and covered by your HMO. Along the way your doctor might discover that you have liver toxicity or drug-induced psychosis from the medicines, and she would treat those complications correctly. You would take almost every single pill for a full year, and in the next few years you would hop into your SUV every now and then for your regular follow-up appointments.

But nine out of every ten human beings in the world aren't lucky. If they get MDR-TB, it may well kill them. They live in places where they can't get the complex diagnostic tests and treatments you would. The drugs and tests, let alone the coordinated care, would be just plain out of reach. They're too poor to have them. In fact, until very recently, the World Health Organization (WHO) thought that the poorest nations on Earth should not even try to use state-of-the-art methods to detect and treat MDR-TB, because they couldn't possibly afford it.

In Carabayllo, things are different. I visited Jessica there last summer and saw it with my own eyes. On Father Jack's church, on the main drag in Carabayllo, is an enormous sign, stretching like a banner across the entire face. It says, "*Sembremos justicia para cosechar amor*": "Let us sow justice to harvest love." Justice means, among other things, that in Carabayllo, if you have MDR-TB you are not excluded from the treatment that can help you just because of where you happen to have been born.

That's because when Father Jack brought Jim Kim and Paul Farmer to Peru, they cooked up a formula for a little justice. Partners in Health came to Carabayllo, as *Socios en Salud,* and began to tackle the "impossible" problem of MDR-TB. People thought they were psychotic, but they went ahead anyway. They set up a local community clinic and they trained a cadre of indigenous health workers—*promotores*—to visit MDR-TB patients in their homes and directly observe every single dose of medication. They worked with the local public health officials to try to find TB cases that were failing treatment so they could detect MDR-TB and individualize treatment plans before it was too late. They bootlegged laboratory services in the United States. They sometimes carried sputum specimens as holy contraband in their own suitcases. They begged, borrowed, and weaseled expensive antituberculosis medications out of their Harvard hospital pharmacies. Eventually, in a really significant victory, they helped to convince the WHO to put the medicines effective against MDR-TB on its model list of essential drugs. When WHO did that, within a few months prices for these drugs on the open market fell by an order of magnitude, so they are now at last within the financial reach of at least some developing nations.

The work of Partners in Health has begun to change mental models worldwide. The main reason is simple: their results are terrific. The findings for the first seventy MDR-TB patients in Carabayllo are impressive: more than 80 percent cured—disease-free. These people started with a disease that is a death sentence in almost all other developing nations.

The cure is spreading. The Ministry of Health in Peru is heading for a nationwide expansion of the Carabayllo program; the WHO has shifted its ground; the prison system in Russia, a hotbed of MDR-TB, is beginning to change its approach; and the same methods of approaching and organizing care may turn out to be effective against AIDS.

It's unbelievable! It makes you wonder. If they can do that there, treat every single MDR-TB case—every single one—in Carabayllo with state of the art care, and promise to leave no one out, what can we do here?

This year, the IHI became the National Program Office for a $21-million project sponsored by The Robert Wood Johnson (RWJ) Foundation, which we call Pursuing Perfection and which Tom Nolan and I direct. Paul and Jim would like this project because it is psychotic, like them. We are trying to find and support a small number of American health care organizations who will join us in our psychosis and try to make the care given in these organizations perfect—all of it— for everyone they serve. RWJ is going to give the six ultimate grantees up to three million dollars and two years to get this job done.

Its original name was the Toyota Project. The theory of social change involved is simple: health care needs a Toyota. The American automobile industry decided to get a lot better in the past two decades—and then did it—for many reasons, but the first reason was that there was a car on the highways—on the American highways—that was astonishingly better than the American cars. In almost all measures of excellence, the Toyota was not just better in 1980 than its American competitors; it was unimaginably better. It took our breath away. Consumers are smart, and so it also took our money away.

The Pursuing Perfection project challenges a few lunatic organizations to try to become America's health care Toyotas, breaking the boundaries of our history and our assumptions. Trying to be perfect.

Of course, three million dollars and two years is nowhere near enough money and time to buy enough straitjackets for these organizations, let alone transform their care. But anyway, we're going for it. We had 226 organizations apply for Pursuing Perfection grants. Our National Advisory Council, which makes the selection, picked twenty-six for site visits last fall, and then picked twelve of them for so-called Phase I planning grants. In March they'll pick six of these twelve for the full two-year grants, and they will be joined by two European teams—from Delft, in the Netherlands, and Jönköping, Sweden. You can follow the project closely on IHI's Web site.

Rather than making them start from scratch, we gave the grantees a running start toward perfection. We recommended a framework for redesigning their organizations, a framework that I think has the potential to support the dramatic new performance levels that we are aiming for in Pursuing Perfection.

I am telling you this because you don't have to have a Pursuing Perfection grant to pursue perfection. You can have the framework, too, for free.

We stole it. The framework comes from the Institute of Medicine's March 2001 report, *Crossing the Quality Chasm: A New Health System for the Twenty-First Century*. The Chasm Report was the final report of the IOM's Committee on the Quality of Health Care in America, better known for its first report, the one on patient safety, called *To Err Is Human*. Although the Chasm Report is less famous, and harder to read, I think it's a much more important document than *To Err Is Human*. In fact, I happen to think it's one of the most important documents in American health care of the past few decades. I think it could do for health care delivery what the Flexner Report did for medical education a century ago. (The Flexner report, issued in 1910, documented the dismal and chaotic state of medical education in the United States, and outlined a radical prescription for its improvement by bringing it firmly into the universities.)

We are suggesting to the Pursuing Perfection sites that the Chasm Report gives them a way to think about what they ought to invent. It's a way to pursue perfection.

Now, the Chasm Report is 335 pages long, and Stephen King did not write it; it is definitely not a page-turner. But it is logical, and I'm going to take a few minutes right now to show you its logic.

The IOM reviewers edited out the most important page in the Chasm Report just before it went to press, but I am here, and they are not, so here it is anyway. This figure shows a hierarchy (Figure 10.1). It segments the health care system into four levels. At the top is the level of purpose—the reason for the system—the aims it serves. At this level, and at this level only, *quality* is defined. Level 1 is the level of the patient and the community, and quality is the degree to which the rest of the system, all the levels, relieve the suffering, reduce the disability, and support the functioning of the patient and community.

The IOM designated six aims for improvement of that work: safety, effectiveness, patient-centeredness, timeliness, efficiency, and equity. *Safety* means not harming patients. *Effectiveness* means stop-

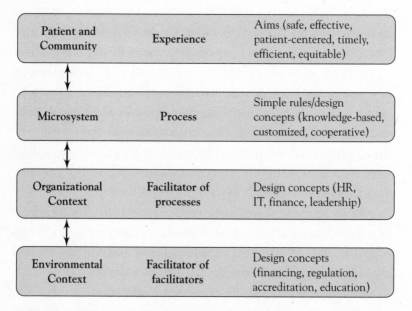

Figure 10.1. The Chain of Effect in Improving Health Care Quality.
Source: Institute for Healthcare Improvement.

ping overuse and underuse—stopping the use of unscientific care and reliably using scientifically proper care. *Patient-centeredness* means giving patients all the information and control they want—offering patients the keys to the car and for those who want them, letting them drive. *Timeliness* means stopping wasting time—stopping all the stupid waiting that everyone—patients, families, and health care workers—has become so used to in health care. *Efficiency* means avoiding waste—of equipment, supplies, capital, ideas, and energy. *Equity* means what Father Jack said—"Sow justice"—although the IOM did not say anything about harvesting love, which may be just as well if you saw the committee.

The Chasm Report makes it clear that health care in America is failing really badly in every single one of these dimensions. It says, "Between the health care we have and the care we should have lies not just a gap but a chasm."

Then the report sounds the following powerful and important warning: "In its current form, habits, and environment, the health care system is incapable of giving Americans the health care they want and deserve. . . . The current care systems cannot do the job. Trying harder will not work. Changing systems of care will."

So, at the other three levels in the model, the Chasm Report asks for changes, big changes. But these are big changes with a compass direction, the one defined at the top level, the level of purpose; true north lies in the improvement of the experiences of patients and communities, and nowhere else. The quality of our care is its capacity to reduce the burden of illness, injury, and disability—nothing else. That's true north.

The second level—Level 2—in the model is the microsystem. This is the term that Paul Batalden and Gene Nelson are teaching us that refers to the small unit that actually does the work—the team of people, along with its local information systems, client populations, space, and work designs—that actually encounters the suffering, the need, and tries to heal. A cardiac surgery team is a microsystem. So is a small office practice, a group of Web page designers, the overnight shift in the emergency department. That's where quality happens or fails—in the work of the microsystem; and the quality—the goodness—of the microsystem is exactly proportional to its ability to reduce the suffering—and nothing else. It's supposed to go true north.

The microsystems are knitted together by organizations—Level 3. The organizations give the microsystems things they can't give themselves—information, financing, architecture, rules, personnel, and so on. Sometimes they work; sometimes they let the microsystems down. This model says that the quality—the goodness—of the organization is the way it helps the microsystems relieve the suffering—and nothing else. True north is absolutely the same direction for organizations as for the microsystems.

And the organizations also have contexts—the broader environment, Level 4, such as health care financing schemes, regulations, accreditation, professional education systems, the tort system, capital markets, and so on. The model says that the quality of the environment is exactly its ability to encourage organizations that help microsystems to relieve suffering—and nothing else. Everybody goes north, or should.

When the Chasm Report says we need changes, it means changes at every one of these levels—aims, microsystems, organizations, and environment. It says we need a new degree of alignment and thinking like a system all along this chain. We need a servant view—all eyes turn north—toward the patient, and all investments are in the relief of pain and the maintenance and restoration of function—to reduce the burden of illness, injury, and disability. Quality is there—and nowhere else. It says we absolutely and always need to remember the people we serve, and we should define our quality consistently, ambitiously, and only in terms of how we are doing for them. Everything else—microsystem designs, organizational forms, organizational survival, social beliefs, laws, regulations, habits—is negotiable, changeable, improvable. I really like that stuff. It sounds right to me.

Now, how are we going to do that? Let's go back to Peru for a minute to look for some ideas. When I visited Carabayllo, I spent my time with Dr. Jaime Bayona, the local hero who combines his vision with Paul Farmer's and Jim Kim's and makes Partners in Health—*Socios en Salud*—work for the people of Lima. Jaime Bayona is quite a guy. I spent a few days with him, visiting clinics and patients and staff. Right away you can sense his dignity, his tirelessness, his humility, his creativity. But the thing that impressed me the most about Jaime as we talked about the patients with MDR-TB, the ones whose lives he is in the process of saving, was this: Jaime Bayona knows their names. All of their names.

We visited a local hospital to see the TB ward. As we walked quietly through it, Jaime pointed out a young doctor in a long white coat who was making rounds with his attending physician. "That's Pedro," Jaime whispered. "He is one of ours." "One of your doctors?" I asked. "Well, yes, now," Jaime answered, "but I mean he was one of our patients. He had MDR-TB."

We had coffee with Pedro—Pedro Huamani, a soft-spoken, shy, smiling young man, unshaven after his night on call—who spoke no English. Through Jaime's translation I heard Pedro's story. He had come from a poor rural area of Peru. He was the first person in his family to reach higher education. Working two jobs, he won his way into the university and medical school. Then he caught tuberculosis. The usual treatment failed, but the local TB program, guided by the old WHO rules, told him he didn't need anything else. So Pedro took his own cultures, did his own sensitivities, and found his own MDR-TB. He found his own death sentence. Still, the routine TB system refused to tackle it. Then Pedro found Jaime. Jaime did not have the funding to support Pedro's treatment, but he took him anyway, against the rules. He cheated a bit to save Pedro's life. He found a way to get medicines to Pedro, keeping only shadow medical records because formal ones could have made for trouble.

Five years later, Pedro is cured, and at the dawn of a professional career. He is thinking of spending it fighting the disease that would, if not for Father Jack, have killed him. Sow justice to harvest love.

I turned to Jaime and asked him, "Do you follow up with your patients? Do you know where they are?"

"Every single one," Jaime Bayona said. "Every single one."

I had heard that phrase once before. It was on a visit with Paul O'Neill at Alcoa. O'Neill was soon to be named Secretary of the Treasury, but on that occasion he was meeting with Maureen Bisognano, Tom Nolan, and me to help us understand the initiative he started in Pittsburgh to drive surgical infections and medication errors to zero in the Pittsburgh area. But O'Neill didn't start by talking to us about perfection in health care. He was too excited about the meeting he had just come from. It was with the principals and superintendent of the schools in Pittsburgh. He challenged them to pursue perfection in education. "Why shouldn't every kid in Pittsburgh read?" he asked. "I told them they ought to make a promise, that every single ten-year-old child in Pittsburgh will read by age ten, one at a time. One at a time," he repeated.

"Every single one"—that's the secret. That's the exact nature of pursuing perfection—in hip surgery or children reading in Pittsburgh, in tackling incurable disease in Carabayllo or in pursuing perfection in American health care. The secret is promising, without compromise, what we will do for each and every person who comes into our care, one at a time.

Look, the Pursuing Perfection Phase I grantees are a great bunch. But they don't have the sole rights to the field of perfection, and the ambition of the IHI isn't at all reserved for them. You can pursue perfection, too. You can play. You are invited to the game. Tell them I invited you. Beat the grantees. You can do it. But you've got to have the password. The password is Jaime Bayona's report and Paul O'Neill's pledge: Every single one. That's how you get into the perfection game.

Let me take the Chasm Report, our new charter document, and see what that would mean. I'd like to try it at Level 2—getting the microsystems right, changing their work so they can do in the future what they cannot now do—improve safety, effectiveness, patient-centeredness, timeliness, efficiency, and equity to unprecedented levels, all together.

The Chasm Report says that microsystem redesign should be guided by ten new "simple rules." You will see here the impact on the IOM of both Tom Nolan and Paul Plsek. Tom taught the IOM committee members about change concepts; Paul taught them about complex adaptive systems. Both of these concepts lead to simple rules—good ideas that the millions of people who work in health care can make into realities by using their imaginations if they get the right support.

The simple rules, ten of them, are supposed to be good notions. They are supposed to offer guidance for change. They are supposed to be better—more powerful—than the prevailing, less effective old rules that run the show now. They are also supposed to be more scientific—more rational.

Here are the rules:

1. *Base care in healing relationships—not visits, as in the current mode.* Give people help through many routes and in many forms, around the clock. Don't rely on the bottleneck of face-to-face visits as the only productive form of care. So if a patient wants to send an e-mail, or talk on the phone, or check the web, don't fight him; help him.

2. *Customize care to the individual patient.* Let's have more variation in response to varying needs. But let's stop the stupid, unscientific, irrational variation in care that seems based on unexamined local habits or some vague sense of the importance of clinical autonomy. We still vary by 50 percent or more in the United States from place to place in the rates of sinus operations, breast cancer surgery, and dozens of other procedures. Let's stop it.

3. *Regard the patient as the ultimate source of control in the system.* Agree that clinicians and institutions can take over control only with the permission of the patient. Not all patients want so

much control, but we should accommodate every single patient's wishes for the degree of control they desire over the decisions that affect them.

4. *Share knowledge and let information flow freely.* We should regard the sharing of information itself as care and healing. Patients should have unfettered access to their own medical records—no permission, fee, or delay. Period. And they should also have easy access to clinical knowledge and scientific resources of any and all types. Whatever they want to know, we should help them learn.

5. *Base decisions on evidence, the best science.* We need to get serious about promising every patient the benefit of care that draws on the best knowledge available anywhere. Put science into practice reliably. Guarantee it. Promise it. We are now just about the only industry in America that basically guarantees its customers absolutely nothing. We don't warrant our work; we should.

6. *Make sure we see safety as a system property, and build patient safety deeply into the designs of care.* Stop relying on exhorting the workforce to give safe care; we have a health care workforce already trying very hard not to harm anyone. We need to make it possible for these good people not to do harm just because they are human. We need to raise respectable and respectful dikes against normal human frailties.

7. *Become transparent.* Anyone who wants it should have information on how well we are doing, on the performance and characteristics of all components of the care system. Cease secrecy as a habit. We need to stop hiding what we do. Don't hide. Disclose.

8. *Anticipate needs rather than mainly reacting.* Stop acting surprised when patients come to us because they are sick. Get ready. Use information, modeling, systems thinking, and scientific designs to make care proactive, agile, and adaptive. Plan our care.

9. *Continually reduce waste in all of its forms, including waste of time, space, ideas, supplies, information, inspections, and spirit.*

10. *Foster cooperation among clinicians and between clinicians and organizations, recognizing cooperation as the highest professional value*

of all. Reduce the suboptimization that comes from thinking and acting in terms of guilds, from organizational and departmental fences, and from social and professional hierarchies.

Three patients are here with me today:

Mrs. Molly Weasley is a forty-two-year-old mother of seven who has just been diagnosed with type 2 diabetes. She has been in good health, except for one episode of reactive depression when her oldest child hijacked a car.

Ron Weasley, her sixth son, has a learning disability and recently broke his right wrist falling off a broom at boarding school.

Mr. Albus Dumbledore is a seventy-eight-year-old chemistry teacher who had one heart attack two years ago, from which he has recovered well—right, Albus? Mr. Dumbledore now has progressive osteoarthritis in his right hip, which limits his walking to two or three city blocks before he has to rest or resort to his broom.

I also have two colleagues with me today: Dr. Donald Olderway and Dr. Donald Newerway. The three of us thought we could illustrate the IOM's simple rules by talking with these three patients, one at a time. As you may have guessed, Dr. Olderway has some real issues with the simple rules.

DR. OLDERWAY: Well, Don, not really issues. Your simple rules sure sound nice. If only health care were that simple; but you and I both know better. You've got to admit the rules are impractical, a little unprofessional—stupid, actually. You'll see.

Okay. Well, Dr. Olderway, where would you like to start? With Mrs. Weasley?

DR. OLDERWAY: So, Molly, I see here that you have diabetes. Diabetes mellitus, type 2. I don't want to you worry too much. We can handle it. Just follow instructions and you'll be fine. Now, let's start with your insulin. What's insulin? Well, Molly, that's a bit hard to explain in lay terms. Your pancreas has some good cells in it that make it, and some bad cells have hurt the good cells, so your pancreas isn't as good as my pancreas. That does not make you a bad person. Here is your insulin prescription. Well, I know you can't read it, Molly; you don't have to. Only the pharmacist does. It says, "Insulin, 31 units. . . ." What's that? It looks like a 2 . . . 21 units? No, it's 31, Molly. Oh, wait a minute, I'll be darned, you're right; it is 21. So, you test your blood sugars at home and call me if things get out of whack. This here is the diet I want you on. Well, I know you like cake, but you'll have to forget it. Trust me. See you next month, Molly. Make an appointment with Sarah on your way out.

Now, Dr. Newerway?

DR. NEWERWAY [on the phone]: Mrs. Weasley, I'm just calling to check up on how you are doing. I've been getting your e-mail questions. Am I answering quickly enough? It sometimes takes my nurse practitioner or me a few hours to get back to you. Thanks, by the way, for helping to work on our diabetes Web site design. Now that you've posted your blood sugar control chart, I've been over it with our chronic care practice team. Is there any chance you'd be willing to come in from time to time to teach some of our newer patients with diabetes about self-care and monitoring at their group visits, or maybe coach them by phone? Yes, I saw that JAMA article last week too. It shows that the blood sugar monitor brand you are on is a little less accurate than the top two brands. I don't think the difference matters, but what do you think? Okay, why don't you stick with your current machine, unless something new pops up about it that concerns you. Our diabetes management team will keep me posted if anything new comes up in the Cochrane Collaborative, AHRQ database, or *Clinical Evidence*. Will you e-mail me if you spot anything I might miss? Thanks.

Cake? You still like the cake. Well, as I've said before, Mrs. Weasley, it's your life, not mine. I am sure you'll make the best decisions for yourself. Eating cake makes some people's blood sugar harder to control, but you know, with your control charts, I bet you'll figure out exactly how to adjust for it. When you do, why don't you make sure to post your comments on the diabetes listserv.

When should you come in again? Oh, I'm not sure, Mrs. Weasley. It's absolutely up to you. With the e-mail, group visits, Web site, and phone, I'm not at all sure you have to come in at all for quite a while, but you're always welcome. Our registry will remind us both when you're due for your next eye and foot exams. You won't get lost, ever. I promise. We guarantee it. Oh, by the way, the registry prompted me to send the computerized prescription to the pharmacy last week. It's a little embarrassing. I goofed. Got your dose wrong as the computer pointed out to me on the spot. It also reminded me to prescribe those special color-coded syringes that you like.

DR. OLDERWAY: You know how much those computers cost?

DR. NEWERWAY [hand over the phone]: Excuse me, Mrs. Weasley. Yup. And I also know how much those computers save. Once we got the costs and the savings onto the same financial statements, they made sense.

One more thing, Mrs. Weasley, if you have the time. Would you mind rating our care in the past month on a scale of one to ten? Thanks. If I could change one thing in my practice next month that would be an improvement from your point of view, what would you suggest?

DR. OLDERWAY: Why are you making more work for yourself? Patients don't really want that much information. They want to think, "Doctor knows best." Anyway, how do you have the time to teach patients all that control chart mumbo jumbo? Besides, it sounds like you're getting a little confused—like between who's the doctor and who's the patient. Remember, you're the one who went to medical school.

Albus, Albus. How nice to see you! How's that hip doing? Pretty sore, huh? I've been telling you, you ought to let Dr. Blarney do his thing and replace it with a nice, new titanium one. Complications? Oh, I don't think so. Well, a few sometimes, but Blarney is the best. Trust me. Things almost never go wrong. I'd hate to see you worrying about it. It'll be on all those permission forms, anyway. And you're fit as a fiddle. The heart attack? What heart attack? Oh, yes, I'm sorry, I forgot about that heart attack. That was while you were away, so I never got the records. Nope, never did. Anyway, we'll take good care of your heart, now that I think of it; we'll get some cardiologist or other to look in on you. Look, any person in their right mind your age ought to have a nice new hip. You can't fly everywhere on that broom of yours. People talk.

DR. NEWERWAY: Mr. Dumbledore, it's so great to see you again. Nice broom. I was reviewing your medical record here on our computer and reminded myself that I should send an e-mail to that cardiologist in San Francisco who did such a good job with your heart attack. I remember how we managed you together that week, and we should let him know how well you've done. Oh, you already have? Oh, here it is. I see you put a note about it right here in your medical record, right here next to the EKG.

DR. OLDERWAY: He *writes* in his medical record?

DR. NEWERWAY: Yeah. He knows stuff.

DR. OLDERWAY: Is that legal?

DR. NEWERWAY: We made it legal.

OK, let's talk about your hip. You have a lot of options, as usual. Can I help you choose? You've been over that CD-ROM on shared decision making in hip replacement. Any questions? Yes, there can be complications. At our hospital, infections are the main ones, which happen in 3.5 percent of cases, with variation among the four surgeons here between 2.5 and 6.5 last year. The surgeon with the highest complication rate turned out to be using a special clamp that was hard to sterilize, so they have that under control, standardized. But here is the outcomes Web page. As you can see, of the five hospitals within fifty miles of here, ours just isn't the safest when it comes to infections right now. Northern Memorial is down below 1 percent, and actually, I'm on the improvement team that's headed there tomorrow to study them. We're also using the surgical simulation lab right now for hip replacement team training, so you'll see our complication rates fall next year. But we did have the highest patient satisfaction last year for hip surgery patients, I think because our rehab education is tops.

Our surgical mortality rate for someone your age is . . . Oh, you don't want to know that? That's fine. Whatever you want. Why don't you and your son play with the outcomes database if you want, and you can see what you think? You'll also find phone numbers of prior patients to call and quiz if you want. I think it'll come down to some slightly better complication rates at Northern, but a little more convenience for your wife and you in travel time here. You'll be the best judge.

What's that? Your wife wants to accompany you right into the operating room and to be in the recovery room when you wake up? Well, of course. Permission? No, Mr. Dumbledore, you don't need my permission or anyone else's for her to be there. We would need your permission if we wanted to separate you, which we don't. You're the boss. Remember, we're guests in your lives.

DR. OLDERWAY: Uh, can I talk with you for a minute? You're asking for trouble again. All that stuff about complication rates—that's an engraved invitation for a lawsuit. Don't you know that if Dumbledore gets an infection, the next call he'll make is to his lawyer? And you just gave him the evidence that your place screws up more than the other.

DR. NEWERWAY: Actually, it's already been in the papers; we put it there. We had a bit of a rough time on the PR front, but we weathered it. Anyway, there is no choice. We've guaranteed total transparency. And even if we didn't tell him in advance about our problems, we'd tell him on the spot. Every time a patient gets injured in care, our hospital says we have to tell the patient, apologize, offer compensation, and if they want it we'll even refer them to a good lawyer. We stand behind our work.

DR. OLDERWAY: I stand behind mine, too. I just don't make my mistakes into front-page news. I don't need to make the lawyers any richer.

DR. NEWERWAY: We have twice as many claims to settle as before, but they settle for 25 percent of the amounts we used to see. It also goes a lot faster, so we've been able to cut our reserves in half. More important, I think the money now goes to injured patients, not to the legal system. And even more important, doctors, nurses, and other staff are speaking up when they see something go wrong.

DR. OLDERWAY: I've never heard anything so naive. It'll serve you right if everyone goes to Northern. Also, those OR nurses are going to love you when the Mrs. comes right into the OR with him. I'd like to see that!

DR. NEWERWAY: We're a team. We had a request like that a year or so ago and we all decided to try it. It worked fine. Our rule is: Patients are the source of control. So, when a patient asks for something, the answer is yes until proven otherwise. We did have one spouse faint, out of over a hundred so far. So we added smelling salts to the room and kept the choice open.

DR. OLDERWAY: So, the inmates are running the asylum. If you're not careful, before you know it they'll be peeing in the staff bathrooms. Just kidding.

Let me talk to the kid.

So, you're Ron. Nice broom, Ron. Broke your arm? Well, no, I didn't know. How would I? Well, Ron, do I work in the emergency department? So, how would I know? Have your mother make an appointment for the cast to come off next week. I've got Thursday at 11 A.M. for cast removals. School? Sorry. You'll have to skip it. I know you'll hate doing that. Can you have a copy of the X-ray? Why? You want to put it on your wall? Right up there with the Grateful Dead? I don't think so, Ron.

DR. NEWERWAY: Hi, Ron. Sure, I saw the emergency room report. We have the same computerized medical record as you do, remember? The same one you can get to from home . . .

DR. OLDERWAY: Kid reads his own medical record?

DR. NEWERWAY: Not often, but it's his. It's about him. We borrow it, but he owns it.

That's why I'm calling you, Ron, just to check in. It'll be time to take off your cast next week. Tell your mom she can bring you in any time she wants; we have open access here. Mark Murray himself taught it to us. You want a copy of your X-ray? To put on your wall? Next to Bono? Sure. What a wonderful idea. It's your picture, anyway, not mine. Can your mom join us for a minute on another extension? Thanks.

Mrs. Weasley, hello again. You can bring Ron in anytime you want next week to have the cast taken off. Just call that morning. Oh, you want to do it yourself? Handy with tools? Okay. That's an interesting proposal. Why not try it, and let me know if you have any questions. I'll talk you through it on an open phone line while you try, and we'll post the test on our Web site afterward. No, I don't have to examine him afterward; let's do that by phone, too. Sound okay? Okay with you, Ron?

Ron, I just wanted to ask you and your mom how things are going at school. How much Ritalin are you taking right now? Ron, can you e-mail me your control chart sometime today? OK, faxing it will be fine. Our cybrarian just let me know that the new

Cochrane Collaborative review of ADD treatment came out yesterday and I want to see if it has any great new ideas for us.

DR. OLDERWAY: Cookbook medicine! Why not use your brain instead of a cookbook?

DR. NEWERWAY: I can't possibly read all the randomized trials. The Cochrane Collaborative does it for me.

I'll have our cybrarian e-mail the Cochrane report to both of you so you can read it, too. Let me know if it gives you any ideas. We can report on it together in our conference call with your teacher, Ron, week after next.

DR. OLDERWAY: Whoa, whoa, whoa. Wait a minute. Did you tell that mom that she can take the kid's cast off herself? That's crazy.

DR. NEWERWAY: Maybe, but it sounds interesting to me. Her hobbies are woodcarving and weaving, Ron's fracture is routine, and I'll be available on the phone if they have any questions. Why waste a visit—for her or for me—if there's a better way? Anyway, who do you think is going to be more careful than his mom in taking off that cast?

DR. OLDERWAY: Sure, let's have everyone take off their own casts. Let's have everyone take out their own stitches. Don, doesn't this sound crazy to you? Talk to the man!

You guys leave me out of this!

DR. NEWERWAY: Absolutely not. I want my care to be customized to every single patient—one at a time. Some patients can take out their own stitches, some can't, some can and don't want to. As far as I'm concerned, every patient is the only patient.

Maybe Dr. Olderway doesn't understand. He can't see how it would be possible to run the show with the new rules. That's partly because of his values. He doesn't really buy the idea of patient-centered, knowledge-based, system-minded care. He thinks . . .

DR. OLDERWAY: Don . . . excuse me for interrupting. You've got it wrong. You're pissing me off.

Can't you see I'm trying to finish my speech here? The play's over.

DR. OLDERWAY: Yeah, but hold on a minute. You make me sound like some kind of creep. Don't you think I have a brain . . . and a heart?

Well . . . yes. Sure. But you're so resistant. I think you're a laggard.

DR. OLDERWAY: Where do you come off saying I don't understand? That I don't see the value of your new rules? I heard your stuff about Jaime Bayona. You know, I used to work in Peru, too. I was in the Peace Corps. I saw those people. I worked every single day for two years to help make their lives better. Hell, I was practically a communist!

Do you think you're the only idealist around here? I wanted to help them; I still do. But do you see the grind I am in every day? More and more forms to fill out. I've been sued twice for mistakes that tear my own heart out. Who has the gall to think they can make me feel guiltier than I already feel or try harder than I already try? Have you ever been sued? You want to encourage patient self-care? One of my partners two years ago told a patient she could take out her own sutures. The wound dehisced and she was awarded $200,000 and the settlement went right into his physician profile.

E-mail care? You've got to be kidding! I'd never get paid, and my medical records committee just sent out a notice that if I tried it I'd have to print out and paste every single e-mail in my office record or they might suspend my staff privileges. I just got a $90 productivity bonus from the same insurance company that won't pay me a nickel for organizing one of your group diabetes visits and won't approve a psych evaluation for a fourteen-year-old patient of mine—Keith (see, I know his name, Keith). I think Keith may be suicidal, and I can't get him help. I'm scared.

Yeah, maybe my old imagination has gone to sleep, Don. Maybe I haven't got the spark I had in the Peace Corps. But don't you think for one minute that I don't care. Maybe while you're preaching about helping the patient—every single one, one at a time—maybe someone ought to think a little about those of us out there helping the patient. What about us? We're the people, too. Every single one. Why don't you sow a little justice *here?*

I guess we owe Dr. Olderway an apology. Maybe he can't buy the future because he has only one way to get there—by stressing the current, familiar designs, and he knows for sure that that won't work. He's been there, done that. So, it seems impossible. Just like international health experts, before Jim Kim and Paul Farmer, knew that people would just have to die of MDR-TB in the poorest nations of the world. It is impossible, without organizations, supportive environments, and great ideas for designs that make new care possible.

Dr. Olderway isn't resisting; he's predicting. If we ask him to do it anyway, without changes that could help him, we are being unjust. It would be like asking the nurses in Carabayllo to cure TB without *Socios en Salud.* Dr. Newerway didn't create success without lots of help. Here is some of the help he got:

- Mark Murray's open access scheduling systems
- Ed Wagner's chronic disease model
- Shared decision-making supports
- A simple, computerized medical record
- Structures for coordinating across boundaries, such as improvement teams and multidisciplinary care teams

- Approaches to advance care planning à la John Wasson—truly managing care proactively, including simple registries, reminder systems, and protocols

- Strong educational supports, technologies, and measurement tools for patient self-care, customized to the needs, desires, and endowments of each individual person

- Senior leaders willing to encourage tests of change in time-honored rules and assumptions, such as those about patient visiting, control over medical records, and access to medical literature

- Knowledge-management systems that put world-class science and evidence at the fingertips of patients and clinicians at the sharp end of care, immediately, with the right kind of library supports and syntheses

- Strong commitments to stratification and segmentation of patient flow, not requiring all patients, no matter what their needs and endowments, to pass through the same nineteenth-century procedural hoops, allowing choices among plausible options, and honoring individual patients' preferences

- Twenty-first-century information technologies, not primarily for the purposes of measuring and judging care, but primarily to put all useful information at the point of care for patients and clinicians to use, on the spot, as they need it

- Unwavering agreement on transparency and disclosure, removing obstacles of local rules, legal fears, and endless signoffs

- Multiple, parallel channels for communication, allowing people in the microsystems to customize what they do, on the spot, to every patient's needs; e-mail, the Web, phone, fax—whatever works, whenever it is needed

- Redefinitions of productivity so that the clinician can focus on healing and knowledge, adjusting work to needs, not subjugating needs to hog-tied work. Providing the freedom to help in the most appropriate way.

I could go on, but you get the idea. New care, supported by new systems. As Bob Waller, former CEO of Mayo Foundation and great friend of the IHI, once said to me, "Everything is impossible, until it's not."

My mind keeps returning to Jim Kim, Paul Farmer, Jaime Bayona, and Carabayllo. The first station on the route to perfection is to believe in perfection. In Carabayllo or Boston, London or Tallahassee, Haiti or Hackensack, only one image of perfection in health care is worthy of us. It is Jaime Bayona's image, which can illuminate the way to cure TB or heal America's care system. "Do you know where they are?" I asked Dr. Bayona. "Every single one," he answered, "every single one."

Father Jack Roussin did not live to see the harvest of the work he began. He died in 1995, of MDR-TB. His banner is still there: "Let us sow justice to harvest love."

And I yield to the temptation to make one more leap with that thought, beyond even pursuing perfection as the aim. To something even bigger.

The shadow of September 11 reaches across time and space into this room at this hour. The world's fear, hate, and grief threaten to dwarf our local tasks and goals, and to make us feel unnecessary. Naturally, then, we, the people, search for connections between what we do and what we want for the world.

Indulge me—how about this: Let us sow justice to harvest love. From the small aim to do well for one patient to the larger one of doing well for all patients, a line leads forward inescapably to justice and to the form of perfection that Jaime Bayona seeks in his work, just as you do in yours. Justice twice: justice for the patient and justice for the people who want to help the patient. Every single ten-year-old will read. Every single tuberculosis victim will get the best chance for life. Every patient is the only patient. Every single doctor or nurse will have a chance to use his or her imagination, to work from the heart, to be understood. To leave no one behind. To leave no one out.

I think this is connected to the deeper issues of our day. I do not for one instant believe that injustice is an excuse for the violence or even for the hatred behind the violence. But I do believe that injustice—exclusion—nourishes hatred.

In its deepest core, the pursuit of perfection is to forget no one. And to forget no one is to pursue justice. And to pursue justice is to pursue love. And to pursue love is to pursue peace. And that is why we are here. Have a wonderful Forum.

Further Reading

Institute of Medicine. *To Err Is Human: Building a Safer Health System.* Washington, D.C.: National Academies Press, 1999.

Institute of Medicine. *Crossing the Quality Chasm: A New Health System for the Twenty-First Century.* Washington, D.C.: National Academies Press, 2001.

11

Plenty

Commentary

Vinod K. Sahney

Donald Berwick asks us to view health care delivery from a new perspective. He asks us to take off the glasses that restrict our view to only one narrow dimension: scarcity. Instead he challenges us to open our minds and take a fresh look at health care delivery from multiple dimensions. Instead of focusing on scarcity of resources, he asks us to examine how to leverage all the resources we already have and begin to utilize their full potential. Berwick recommends that we examine four valuable resources that are in abundant supply: patients and their families, employees, knowledge, and global brains.

Patients and their families. In most health care systems, the patient is viewed as someone to whom to provide care—rarely as an active partner managing his or her care. What if we changed our thinking and considered multiple ways to partner with patients? Patients could help us improve processes of care, assist us in defining their specific needs, monitor their own care, and even provide some of their own care.

Other industries have changed their processes to involve customers as key partners in processing work. Examples abound in airlines, grocery chains, and package shipping, to name a few. E-tickets now account for the majority of airline tickets used in this country.

Travelers can log in, view different schedules, select and book flights, and get boarding passes—without ever speaking to airline personnel. Involving customers has reduced the cost of processing a ticket from more than ten dollars to less than ten cents, converting a costly process for the airlines into a relatively inexpensive one, with higher customer satisfaction.

What if we let patients book their own appointments, fill out a preliminary history before seeing their physician, monitor their own vital signs, and use the Internet to communicate with their physicians? We would suddenly have additional resources—and more satisfied patients.

Employees. Organizations typically view their front-line employees as providing bodies and hands to do the work. Employees are supposed to do what they have been told to do. What a waste! Health care employees are highly educated. They include nurses, pharmacists, respiratory therapists, and many other trained caregivers with college educations. What if we changed our paradigm to one in which every employee has two jobs: first, the job they were hired to do; second, and more important, improving the process by which they are currently performing their job.

Nelson and colleagues recently published an article on what makes front-line care delivery teams produce exceptional quality of care. They call these systems of care at the front line *microsystems*. They conclude that nine characteristics distinguish successful microsystems: leadership, culture, organizational support, patient focus, staff focus, interdependence of care team, information and information technology, process improvement, and performance patterns. Successful care delivery systems involve their employees through an environment that encourages and supports them in using their intellectual abilities to improve care.

Knowledge. Opening our minds to knowledge allows us to learn from others and improve care. We need to create an environment in every microsystem of care that allows us to view the performance of the system over time. Berwick refers to the classic work of George Box and William Hunter, who use a technique called *evolutionary process improvement.* By making planned changes to the process and studying the impact of those changes, we can learn as well as continuously improve the processes while delivering care.

Global brains. Health care systems are saddled with the "NIH syndrome": Not Invented Here. Berwick challenges us to look for ideas outside our organizations, not only in the United States, but worldwide. We should actively look for good ideas and, if we find one, be the first one to steal it and implement it. The Institute for Healthcare Improvement has developed a specialized process called the Breakthrough Series to mine good ideas from large numbers of sources in a systematic manner and help organizations implement those ideas. Breakthrough Series collaboratives have been conducted in such areas as ICU, ER, waits and delays, supply chain, and chronic diseases. In every case, we have found that no single organization has all of the good ideas. Learning from others helps us to leverage the improvement process within our own organizations.

Once again Berwick has challenged us to think differently. Instead of citing scarcity as the reason for not providing great care, he challenges us to recognize and leverage our existing resources to take our health care systems to new heights of efficiency and effectiveness.

Reference

Nelson, E. C., and others. "Microsystems in Health Care: Learning from High-Performing Front-Line Clinical Units." *Joint Commission Journal on Quality Improvement*, 2002, 28(9), 472–497.

Plenty

14th Annual National Forum on Quality Improvement in Health Care

Orlando, Florida, December 10, 2002

M y good friend Paul Batalden founded the Institute for Health-care Improvement (IHI). He was our first board chair.

Paul is a lunatic. He drives me crazy. The way he does that is this: every so often he says something very weird, which then rattles around in my head for years, the way the song "Hey There, Georgie Girl" once did for ten or twelve weeks.

For example, here is something Paul said about three years ago that I haven't been able to get out of my mind. He said, "We should work not from an assumption of scarcity, but from an assumption of abundance."

See what I mean?

Hey, Paul, you're a lunatic. Haven't you heard of the Balanced Budget Amendment? The nursing shortage? The workforce cutbacks in health care? Don't you know that hospitals are losing money, patients are losing insurance, doctors are losing morale? Scarcity is everywhere, Paul: no prescription drug benefit, poor information technology and not enough capital to buy more, gaps in leadership, gaps in coverage, gaps in measurement, gaps in quality—a gap so wide that the Institute of Medicine calls it a chasm.

So why can't I get the idea out of my head? An assumption of abundance. By the way, this idea also appears in Steven Covey's book, *The Seven Habits of Highly Effective People*.[1]

Keynote speech presented at the 14th Annual National Forum on Quality Improvement in Health Care, Orlando, Florida, December 10, 2002.

Our Forum theme this year is "Movement." Move, moving, movement. Mass in motion, momentum.

It's a pun.

Our work together on improvement must now become a movement—*has* become a movement. We want to say we have enough momentum now to get the job done. And people in movements need to believe something together. Not something rigid, but something sustaining. You know what a movement needs? It needs optimism.

"An assumption of abundance." Now, wouldn't that be nice?

This year my wife introduced me to the work of Amory Lovins, founder and head of the Rocky Mountain Institute and one of the leading thinkers in the environmental movement. I'm only going to scratch the surface of Lovins' work. You can find more at www.rmi.org or in his book coauthored with Paul Hawken and L. Hunter Lovins, *Natural Capitalism*.[2] Like Batalden, Lovins is a lunatic. He believes in abundance when most people around him can see only scarcity.

Lovins and his coauthors show a diagram of a large rectangle with a small circle inside it. Suppose I tell you that one of these—the circle or the rectangle—is the human economy—all of it—and the other is the environment. But I don't tell you which is which. So, which is which?

Everybody gives the same answer. It's obvious. The economy sits inside the environment, not the other way around.

In fact, the environment is the main supplier to the economy. It allows the economy to exist. The universe gives the economy its energy—light and heat. It supplies the raw materials—renewable ones, such as trees, and nonrenewable ones, such as metal ores—all the raw materials, for everything. The environment provides services too—it removes wastes, purifies water, recycles carbon, and also provides human cultures, beliefs, and behaviors.

Now, Lovins and his coauthors called their book, *Natural Capitalism*. Classical capitalism recognizes three kinds of resources for the economy of production: human capital, financial capital, and manufactured capital (infrastructure, machines, and so on). But Lovins and his coauthors argue that there is a fourth input; they call it *natural capital*. They argue that the stuff nature supplies to the economy dwarfs the other three kinds of resources.

A smart capitalist—a successful capitalist—they say, doesn't waste resources. That's a way to go out of business. So, they ask, how smart are we?

They analyze the automobile. The purpose of a car, let's say, is to move people from one place to another. If we say that a car consumes one hundred units of energy, converting it into heat, light, and changes in momentum, how many of those units actually are getting the job done—moving human beings? The answer is one. When a car burns fuel, 80 percent of the energy is lost in heat; only 20 percent turns the wheels. Ninety-five percent of the weight the wheels move is the car—only 5 percent is the driver. Five percent of 20 percent is 1 percent. The rest of the energy conversion is waste—99 percent is waste.

Here's another example. The economy of the United States converts lots of things into other things—ore into metal, metal into shapes, shapes into refrigerators. So, you can imagine our economy as a big conversion chain for materials. So, here's a question. For each person in America—average weight, say, 120 pounds—how many pounds of materials does our economy process each year? The answer is one million pounds. For every person in this room, every year, one million pounds of something is made into something else. And then we throw almost all of the one million pounds away.

Here's a partial inventory of what America throws away every year:

- 3.5 billion pounds of carpet landfill

- 3.3 trillion pounds of carbon in carbon dioxide emissions

- 19 billion pounds of polystyrene peanuts

- 28 billion pounds of discarded food in homes

- 360 billion pounds of organic and inorganic chemicals used in processing

- 710 billion pounds of hazardous waste from chemical production

- 3.7 trillion pounds of construction debris

Let's look at that list and ask, How do we get to do that? Where do we get the stuff to waste in the first place? What gives us the chance to make it and throw it away? It wasn't any of the first three forms of capital: people, money, or machines. The chance to throw so much away comes from a different supplier: nature.

The estimated economic value of the ecosystem's input to the world's economy is $36 trillion a year. The world's total gross domestic product is $39 trillion a year. If you look at the $36 trillion as income on capital assets, the ecosystem's capital value is between $400 trillion and $500 trillion.

So why don't we see it that way? Lovins and his coauthors say we don't see the value of natural capital because we attribute to it a particular price: zero. We don't count it, so we don't know it. It is inexhaustible, anyway, isn't it? There's no charge.

Of course, one of the central concerns of the environmental movement is that nature's capital may not be inexhaustible; it may be limited. We can use it up like we can use up a bank account or a machine. We just don't know it because no banker tells us. So we deplete natural capital. In the past thirty years we've used up one-third of our planet's total natural wealth. A fourth of the earth's topsoil is gone in the past half-century; so is a third of its forests. We're losing fresh water ecosystems at 6 percent per year, marine life at 4 percent per year.

That's big trouble, but it's not what I want to focus on this morning. This is a long way around to health care, but I want to think with you instead about what happens if we ask Lovins' questions not about the environment but about another corner of the world that we care about—the struggle against disease, the pursuit of health. Let's take a look again at Lovins' diagram: a small circle inside a big rectangle.

Suppose I tell you that the circle is health care—our hospitals, clinics, doctors, nurses, staff, managers, physical plants, machines, and processes. What, then, is the rectangle? In what are we embedded? What, to stretch the question further, is our supplier? What is the "natural capital" of health care—important, maybe immense, essential, looming, there before us and after we are gone, crucial, but maybe, like air and water, unpriced? Invaluable but unvalued? Could that be what Paul Batalden means by *abundance*?

You see, if we could find the abundance, we could ask the same questions that Lovins and his coauthors ask: What do we waste? What comes to us in such plenty that we cannot see it? That we make its apparent price zero? And in not seeing it and not valuing it, is it possible that, as with clean air and good soil, we slowly, insidiously, and unconsciously deplete it? Starving for resources, is it possible that we throw away the biggest resources we have?

A movement would think differently. A movement might say, "Look, everybody. Look what we found. Plenty." The environmental movement says, "Look, everybody, we found a rich and generous earth." The feminist movement says, "Look, everybody, half of humankind bottled up by gender prejudice." The civil rights movement finds abundant talent and spirit wasted by racial prejudice.

We are going to have to look pretty hard in health care for a sense of plenty. We're so far down the road of an assumption of scarcity. Our lobbyists lobby in Washington and in the state houses for more and more. Our professionals feel drained by demands on their time and energy. Our patients and their advocates stand guard lest something be withheld. The movie *John Q* is a box office smash.

Can I tell you a story?

Jim Lang is a computer systems manager in Cincinnati. He has two children with cystic fibrosis (CF): Alicia, who is eleven, and Nick, who is eight. I met Jim during a site visit to Cincinnati Children's Hospital, which is participating in the IHI-Robert Wood Johnson Foundation Pursuing Perfection project.

Cincinnati Children's Hospital invited Mr. Lang to keynote our site visit. Here is how he started his speech: "It is May 4, 2008, two o'clock in the morning. It's eighteen hours before Alicia's senior prom. She has been coughing most of the night and she comes into our room and says she can't sleep. She's having trouble breathing. She has tears in her eyes and she's having chest pains. Her face is turning blue and she's coughing up blood."

Mr. Lang is a computer systems engineer, but he doesn't see that anymore as his job. He says, "My job is to find a cure for my kids by the time Alicia is driving and Nick is a teenager, and to keep them as healthy as possible until a cure is found. But," he says on our site visit, "to get my job done right, I need your help."

Believers in scarcity tell Jim Lang this: "Gee, Jim, we'd love to help you. But you need to understand *our* problem. We're just strapped. Really tired. Our budget's very tight. Medicaid reimbursements are down. We're short nurses, and the HMOs are watching every penny. We'd love to help, Jim, but times are tough."

Jim isn't buying it. He puts hundreds of hours a year into helping his kids live—he says, "I quit figuring when I got over two thousand hours." Now he serves on Cincinnati Children's CF Quality Initiative Core Team. But in his speech he said, "I am not here to waste my time! I keep coming back because I want to do everything I can so that on May 4, 2008, at two o'clock in the morning, Alicia won't need to wake me up."

Everyone in this room knows that if Jim's job is to help his daughter, our job is to help Jim. Period. All 3,500 of us work in health care for one reason only—same as Jim—to make Alicia's senior prom night romantic. And in pursuit of that aim—in pursuit of perfection, a perfect night at the prom—arguments from scarcity just won't do. They are not right. They cannot be right. We cannot let them sound right. Not "Sorry, Jim, we can't" but "Of course, Jim, we will." That's our movement.

In our movement we are going to find the wealth, not complain about the poverty. We are going to work from an assumption of abundance, not an assumption of scarcity.

What, then, do we have in abundance? Four things at least, as plentiful, if we can harness them, as sunlight, air, and water, but as exhaustible—to our surprise—if we are so foolish as to value them at zero.

First, there is Jim Lang himself.

The patient and the family are natural capital. We cannot afford to waste them. I feel, with great frustration and frankly a little anger, that our talk nowadays—widespread, politically correct, almost ritual—about patient-centeredness is actually only a pale image of what we should mean—can mean. Our rhetoric is fraudulent. And our choices are wasteful.

Ken Greenberg is a skilled historian and now a filmmaker on the team of award-winning filmmakers who are documenting the work of the hospitals and health plans involved in the Pursuing Perfection project—bold, courageous, inspiring places that are seeking to become the Toyotas of health care.

As part of their charter in this project, all of these sites—Cincinnati Children's Hospital included—are pledging to become patient-centered, in the spirit of the Institute of Medicine's *Crossing the Quality Chasm* report.

But with their eyes as artists, social scientists, and unbiased outside observers, Ken Greenberg and his filmmaker colleagues are returning from days and days at these struggling sites with the hard-hitting report that they are not in fact patient-centered; that they are not even close. Ken tells me that he now thinks the true meaning of patient-centeredness—the right meaning—is fundamentally subversive to our traditions. It involves nothing less than the overthrowing of an old order. But on the other side of that transition lies abundance.

Here is the abundance we do not yet see: patients and their families bring to us, without fee or charge, their lives. Jim Lang wants to help us help him to help his children. Everything he knows, everything he experiences, everything he can do is at our disposal and theirs. Patients and families bring to us their expertise, their commitment to themselves, their love of each other, their houses, their gardens, their hobbies, and most of all their innate, natural capacities to heal. Nature has spent 3.8 billion years of R&D developing biological healing capacity, and it walks into our doors—free, for nothing—wanting to help get done what we are trying to get done—survival, healing. The selfish gene wants to work for us.

What do we do with this gift? We discard it, ignore it, dismiss it, disable it, demote it, demean it, silence it, confine it.

I can't resist telling you about Steve Bertrand—he's called Bert. He is the owner of Bertrand Hydraulics in Green Bay, Wisconsin. More to the point here, Bert is, in fact, the chairman of the rules committee of the U.S. Lawn Mower Racing Association. It has 750 members in twenty-two states. Their Web site is www.letsmow.com.

These 750 people race lawn mowers—riding mowers, Bert clarified. They race in four classes, but all on stock mowers, the kind you find at Sears or John Deere stores. They can't change the engine or the chassis or the wheels, although U.S. Lawn Mower Racing Association (USLMRA) rule VII-A is quite sensible: no blades.

A Sears riding mower, model 27191, with a twenty horsepower V-Twin cylinder Briggs and Stratton overhead valve engine and a forty-two-inch EZ3 grass-cutting deck, is advertised to run at a top speed of 5.2 miles an hour. Guess how fast Steve Bertrand can make it go in a USLMRA race? I'll give you a hint: last year Bert placed thirteenth in Class B nationally; his son placed fifth.

The answer is sixty-two miles an hour. Without blades. These people can get sixty-two miles an hour out of your lawn mower. Talk about abundance. Talk about movement!

I asked Bert how you make a 5.2-mile-an-hour machine go sixty-two. Basically, you switch the front belt from stock 4 inches to

7½ inches, and the stock rear belt from 9 inches to 3 inches. That takes you from a gear ratio of 3:1 to 10:1 or so. Then you take the governor off the engine so its maximum 3,600 rpm limit goes to 7,000. Then you do a bunch of other stuff that I can't even begin to understand, much less explain. And by the way, you take the blades off—duh.

Bert has been at this for ten years. He loves it; he's good at it.

Now, put Bert into a hospital. Put him in a johnnie so his underwear shows. Label his arm. Talk at his bedside as if he weren't there. Put it in Latin. Tell him the visiting rules: he takes his own pills at home, but not here. Instead, take his pills away, and then use your own in a little paper cup and dole them out to him four times a day. If he asks for his laboratory result, tell him you need permission to show it to him, because the numbers might scare him—the numbers might scare the thirteenth fastest lawn mower rider in America. Yell out "Bert" in the waiting room, but introduce yourself as "Dr. Jones," or not at all. Keep him waiting. Keep him guessing. Make him tell you his name, address, and phone number five times; make him tell his symptoms ten times. Take his blood pressure twenty times without ever telling him what it means. Hurt him with an error, but never tell him, because he might be angry.

Make noise. Lots of noise—24/7. Wake him three times a night and at 6 A.M. rounds. Clang the cart, beep the beepers, laugh in the corridor. Feed him, but not according to his nature. When he asks for a snack at night, tell him the kitchen is locked, or bring him a slice of white bread. Make the smells strange, the lights harsh, the bed mechanical, the night lonely, the day boring. Do not ask Bert for his opinion, or his help, or his preferences, or his values, or even his knowledge of himself.

In short, tell Bert, regarding the lifetime and skills and wisdom and special knowledge and dexterity and friends and neighbors he brings to us—tell him, "No thanks, Bert. We'll take over."

Bert can make a lawn mower go sixty-two miles an hour. Can you? Well, no. But what does that have to do with anything?

Everything. Patients bring us wealth and we make it slag. Patient-centeredness means valuing everything—everything—that the patient, the family, and the community bring into the struggle against disease—the struggle for health. It means using the natural capital of natural healing. We are not authentically patient-centered until we have wasted none of it. Amory Lovins and his coauthors call it *radical resource productivity*. They have designed a car that gets ninety-nine miles per gallon and that costs not a nickel more than the car you drive now.

I suggest that we have a long, long way to go. I suggest that Ken Greenberg is right. When we really become patient-centered, it will feel utterly subversive. We will have overthrown a basic belief system and abandoned a raft of deeply embedded habits about who in health care has what to contribute to whom. That's one version of the circle and the rectangle; the circle is our work, the rectangle is the lives, communities, talents, and world of our patients, in which our efforts are embedded and which can, if we will let them, be suppliers of extraordinary value. I said it last year and the year before and I'll say it again: We are not hosts to our patients, we are guests in their lives. When we get that straight we will begin to see the abundance in what they bring to us.

Cincinnati Children's Hospital is trying now not to waste that resource. They cannot afford to. Jim Lang is on the team. When other supplies are scarce, they need to use what is abundant. Terri Schindler, a CF nutritionist at Cincinnati who also has a teenage daughter with CF, coleads the CF team. She writes to me, "My daughter, who likes to be independent, is now allowed to draw her own blood through the port—never misses." When her daughter had surgery, Terri was allowed to be at her side in the recovery room before she was fully awake. "It was hard to arrange," Terri says, "but it was a step in the right direction." I, of course, look forward to when no mother ever has to tell us that being at her child's side was "hard to arrange," or when taking care of oneself to the full extent of possibility is not something we have the temerity to believe we are entitled to "allow."

Last month, the hospital launched a test in which patients and families, not staff, designed the care plans in routine CF admissions— when the respiratory therapy treatments are given and when patients get their antibiotics. The result so far is what I would expect: better care plans, easier to implement, far more efficient. That's because the best experts on each patient—the patient himself or herself and loved ones—are "allowed" to be the experts that they are. I personally hope that Cincinnati takes the next logical step soon, at least as a trial, inviting patients and families to run the CF unit for a while and make any changes they wish.

Now, the way that Cincinnati Children's is actually making these changes draws on the second form of abundance—the talents and spirits of their own employees.

Take, for example, Maria Britto. Maria is an adolescent medicine doctor in the CF unit. I've seen her there and I know she represents abundance. You can see it in her eyes—intense, honest, thoughtful, open, committed to Jim Lang and his kids without the slightest doubt in the world. She is not alone. I see it in Jim Acton, head of the CF Center and Terri's coleader of the improvement team. I see it in the staff, who join with them in the pursuit of perfection.

What lies within the workforce of health care is exactly the same form of wealth that Jim Lang offers: the experience of their whole lives. What Maria, Jim, and their colleagues (the doctors, nurses, pharmacists, therapists, managers, receptionists—the workforce) bring to their work has nothing to do with a time clock. They bring their entire selves. And on the whole we waste it.

To recognize that abundance, we will have to leave behind as soon and as clearly as we can the legacy of Frederick Taylor and the view that workers are *hands* rather than *minds*.

Henry Ford and Frederick Taylor were able to put a Model-T Ford in every middle-class garage because they abandoned craftsmanship in favor of what Taylor called *scientific management*, by which he meant the new craft of standardizing work. By designing and then strictly enforcing work procedures, he could ensure that a workforce that made axles and wheels would make all axles identical and all wheels identical, and that then allowed very rapid assembly of cars from bins of parts. The results were speed, quality, and efficiency that were never seen before the era of mass production.

The hidden cost, of course, was to the human spirit. Workers had to become "hands" because their minds would screw up the process. An inventive worker—one who thought too hard—would make weird axles and nonconforming wheels, and the assembly line would grind to a halt. Frederick Taylor knew absolutely that the human spirit requires an opportunity to think, learn, and invent, and he really did want workers to do all of those things—but he wanted them to do those things at home in their leisure time, not at work. Design belonged in the design shop. To work was to follow rules, not to make rules. Certainly not to break rules.

Health care has taken a century to learn how badly we need the best of Frederick Taylor. If we can't standardize appropriate parts of our processes to absolute reliability, we cannot approach perfection. So we have become very interested in guidelines, protocols, and standards so we can be reliable. Blair Sadler and his colleagues at San Diego Children's Hospital have shown brilliantly how much can be achieved, financially and clinically, when a culture adopts the wisest forms of evidence-based standards.

But our love affair with Frederick Taylor is risky; we can overshoot. If we write too many manuals, if we standardize the wrong parts of our care, we are going to drive the spirit out of the workforce in our attempt to drive reliability into it. The secret lies in balancing wise standardization with even wiser invitations. We need to ask the workforce to redesign its work. We need to invite Maria Britto and Jim Acton to use their whole selves to make their work together better and better.

They want to do it. The people who give health care can and will reinvent the care if they are invited authentically to do so.

You can see it at Cincinnati. Maria and Jim have now defined *improvement* as part of their jobs. Their senior leaders give them the time, the encouragement, and the safety to design and redesign CF care, from the ground up, with patients and families as their colleagues—no, not as their colleagues, but as their bosses.

Here is what it looks like. Let me show you a little project done by another physician at Cincinnati Children's—John Bucuvalas. The leaders there told John that his mind counted, not just his hands. He got to enroll in Brent James's Advanced Training Program, spending four weeks in Salt Lake City, supported by his hospital. They put him in charge of a medication safety team. John is a gastroenterologist involved in liver transplantation and he was concerned about the costs and hazards of new antirejection drugs, such as tacrolimus—a very powerful, expensive, and potentially dangerous drug. He learned that twelve months after transplantation, barely half of the tacrolimus drug levels were in the safe and proper range. John developed a simple statistical process control chart method, involving patients and nurses directly in monitoring the levels, and in short order had seventeen out of nineteen levels in tight and efficient control. Here is what happened for one little girl, for example, as her levels came right into line with that intervention (Figure 11.1).

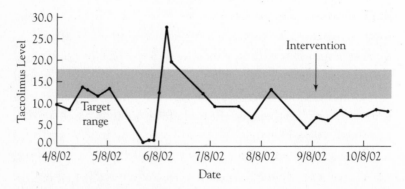

Figure 11.1. Tacrolimus Blood Levels: Movement Toward a Stable Process.
Source: John Bucuvalas, Cincinnati Children's Hospital.

When I ask people like John why he is doing this, I always—always—get the same answer. His colleague, a surgeon named Fred Ryckman, put it this way: "It's because every single day I go to work, I want the people I help to have the same experience I would want for my spouse, my parent, my child, or myself." You can believe him or not. I do.

That will to excellence is present everywhere in health care. It doesn't come from professional training. It doesn't come from professional ethics. It doesn't come from that little circle. It comes from the great big rectangle of our lives. The will to do well—the quest for pride, the joy of achievement, the warmth of serving—these are natural capital, human traits. Not of all human nature, not all the time, but enough, plenty enough. We can waste them and we can deplete them. It is possible, if we try hard enough, to make Maria Britto and John Bucuvalas *not* care. But at the start the will to have pride in work is not scarce; it is everywhere abundant. Don't be fooled by the technique. What John Bucuvalas and his colleagues did for tacrolimus levels (fundamentally improve care) can be done by anyone who can draw a graph over time—and that is nearly anyone at all. This and hundreds of other improvements can be done thousands and thousands of times by thousands and thousands of people if we invite them, encourage them, help them, and teach them. It is exactly what they want to do with their lives. In an important way, it's exactly the same reason that Steve Bertrand wants to drive a lawn mower at sixty-two miles an hour.

If 750 people want letsmow.com, how many might like letshelpJimLang.org?

But neither Jim Lang's skill nor Maria Britto's commitment is enough. To realize their potential, they must have knowledge. Jim Lang must know how to keep prom night happy, and Maria Britto must know how to help him do it.

And here is the third abundance: we *have* the knowledge. It's just tricky to find it, because a lot of it comes in disguise—the disguise of the variation among us. The largest R&D laboratory in

American health care is American health care itself. Every day we
are engaged in an immense uncontrolled experiment—in five thousand hospitals and a hundred thousand offices, housing a vast collection of different, potentially informative ways of working.

George Box has said, "Every process produces information on
the basis of which it can be improved." But to hear the lessons, we
must listen.

But we don't often listen. Just as we too often tell Jim Lang to
remain quiet and tell Maria Britto to read the manual, we too often
throw away the lessons from the variation we could observe. We pay
the tuition but we never take the course.

It happens for many reasons, but the biggest one is fear.

In the past year, the IHI was blessed to have Professor Brian Jarman as a senior fellow in our offices. Brian is the leading general
practitioner in the United Kingdom; he just retired as professor and
chair of general medicine at Imperial College and St. Mary's Hospital. In a few months he'll become the next president of the British
Medical Association. He is a world-class clinician and a world-class
epidemiologist. For many years he's worked with large databases in
the United Kingdom, studying standardized in-hospital mortality
rates. Now Brian is working with large American databases, such as
Medicare's Medpar data, and he's worked out models for assessing
hospital-specific standardized mortality rates for American hospitals.

Here is a scatterplot of 250 random hospitals, in this case using
Agency for Healthcare Research and Quality Hospital Care and
Utilization Project data (Figure 11.2). It looks the same as the scatterplot for Medicare data, which is all in the public domain. You
can have it any day you want it.

The vertical axis shows hospital standardized mortality rates. Each
dot is a hospital and each hospital's rate is adjusted here for many,
many potentially confounding variables—both patient factors, such as
diagnosis, age, sex, and source of admission; and hospital and community variables, such as workforce ratios, size, hospice availability,
and so on. On this vertical scale, one hundred is by definition the

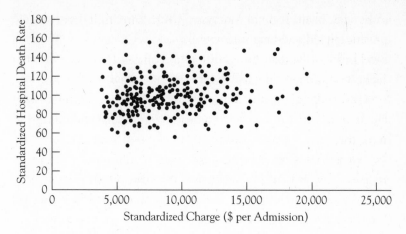

Figure 11.2. Hospital Death Rate Versus Charge per Admission.
   Note: Death rate standardized for age, sex, race, payer, admission, source, and type; charge per admission standardized for age and diagnosis.
   Source: Agency for Healthcare Research and Quality, 1997 data.

adjusted death rate for an average American hospital. So, a dot at seventy, for example, is a hospital with an adjusted death rate 30 percent below the average, and a hospital at 130 is 30 percent above the average. Get it?

The horizontal scale is the same sort of adjusted number for the hospital's average charge per case. If you use data for Medicare reimbursement or for actual costs, you get the same answer.

What do you see here? On the vertical scale, mortalities in this sample range from about 40 to about 160—that's a 400 percent range in the chances of dying. On the horizontal scale, the range is about 500 percent—from $4,000 per case to $20,000 per case—in what the hospital got paid, on average.

Data such as these are scary. In fact, people—especially clinicians and hospital leaders—who see the data always go through some kind of Kübler-Ross death-and-dying stages.

Stage one is this: *"The data are wrong."* So there are lots of questions about adjustments, hidden variables, poor input information, and so on. Brian Jarman has heard these for many years, and he continually adjusts and improves his model. Brian has met with many of his colleague epidemiologists of the first caliber through the years. He has worked for hours on end to make the model better. He has gone into real hospitals and studied the quality of the data he is using. You can believe me or not—it's your choice—but here's the deal: Brian's findings may not be perfect, but in my view they are plenty good enough to act on.

Stage two is this: "OK, *the data are right, but it's not a problem.*" You know the bumper sticker: "Stuff happens." Variation in outcome is part of the game. This is just the hard reality. People die. Mistakes happen. American health care isn't perfect, but it's the best in the world. Yadda, yadda, yadda. Go away, Brian, leave me alone.

Stage three is this: "OK, OK. *The data are right, and it is a problem. But it's not* my *problem.*" I didn't do it. The dog ate my homework. CMS (Centers for Medicare & Medicaid Services) made me do it. The lawyers made me do it. Management made me do it. Or worst excuse of all, the patients made me do it.

Abundance people are in stage four—the data are good enough, it is a problem, it is our problem, and we intend to do something about it. In stage four, people who look around for ways to make things better are going to find some answers—or at least some darn good questions—right in front of their faces. Look back at Brian's scatterplot. There—down there—in the lower left-hand corner. Jewels. Diamonds. Abundance. Hospitals—for real—with apparent standardized death rates one-fourth of the highest, purchased by CMS or Medicaid or General Electric, or you, for one-fifth of the price of the highest. Who are those guys? And is there a chance they could help us all?

To help our movement, IHI has started a new network called IMPACT, which now has almost ninety hospitals and clinics in it. But I'll warn you that you have to be at stage four to make it worth your while to join. Of course, I know that you are going to have to go through stages one, two, and three first. So I encourage everyone to go through them. Please do; be my guest. Deny, justify, and blame—in that order. Please. Just do it really fast, so we can get to work together.

Practically no one in health care knows their own hospital's standardized mortality rate, much less the name and location of the lower left-hand corner places. But a few do know. They are in the IMPACT network, so they saw their own data. One such group found out that their mortality rates vary by 40 percent. They know that on the average they're 30 percent above the national average. Then, instead of throwing the jewels away, their CEOs met with Brian Jarman, learned what he knew, and started together to try to understand it. They have decided to change it. They are going to move their dot. They have decided to go wherever they can to get better ideas for care—and they might start with the lower left-hand corner. Other groups have done the same.

Let me show you some of their recent work—hot off the presses. A lot of the IMPACT hospitals have been studying and sorting fifty deaths each into four boxes, in a model thought up by Tom Nolan (Figure 11.3):

Box A: Patients who had been admitted for comfort care only but who were admitted to the ICU—5 percent

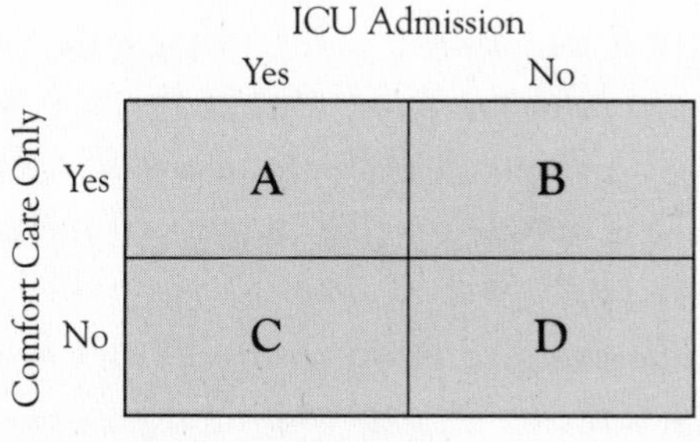

Figure 11.3. Analyzing Hospital Data.
Source: Institute for Healthcare Improvement.

Box B: Patients admitted for comfort care who were admitted to the hospital wards—25 percent

Box C: Patients admitted to the ICU for treatment—not comfort care—35 percent

Box D: Patients admitted to the regular floors for treatment but who died on the same admission—35 percent

Each box contains lessons and opportunities for process improvement. Box A raises questions about inappropriate use of the ICU and the capacity of the hospital to offer hospice care. Box B raises questions about the hospital's excellence in end-of-life care and about community resources that would make hospitalization unnecessary. Box C raises questions about state-of-the-art care in the ICU. And Box D is about unexpected deaths—surprises—and the hospital's ability to triage and respond to emergencies.

These hospitals—and more than eighty others in our IMPACT network—are my heroes. They are after radical resource productivity. They recognize abundance. They convert fear to process thinking. They convert variation into knowledge. They're at stage four. They refuse to discard opportunity into a black hole of denial, ignorance, or apathy. They don't think that denial, justification, or blame are very good plans for getting Alicia to the prom.

Bob Waller—former CEO of Mayo Foundation and current IHI board member—asked me rhetorically, by the way, which is worse, ignorance or apathy. His answer to his own question was profound: "I don't know, and I don't care."

Here's how it works for our boss, Jim Lang. The Cystic Fibrosis Foundation collects nonidentifiable patient-level information on a voluntary basis from the 160 CF care centers in the United States, creating an annual database on care and outcomes. It analyzes these data and feeds back the results as percentile scores to each CF center. That's how Cincinnati Children's Hospital knows that it has some improvement to do in its nutritional care of its CF patients—they are at the forty-fifth percentile nationally—and in preservation of lung function they are at the thirtieth percentile nationally.

Now, you might wonder how I could let this cat out of the bag. How could I show you publicly the relative performance of the Cincinnati Children's CF program? The answer is that Cincinnati Children's has *already* let the cat out of the bag. They told their own patients—in fact, their own local press—exactly where they rank. Then they promised to improve—dramatically—fast.

The best way to start doing that is pretty clear—at least it is to me, and to them. Find the best and see what they are doing differently. So they asked. They asked the CF Foundation to tell them the names of the best hospitals in nutrition and lung function preservation.

Now comes the hard part of the story. It isn't so easy to mine this gold. It is against CF Foundation policy to reveal the names of the centers in the rankings. There are some good reasons for caution. Public release of the results would scare some hospitals. Others would misuse it for competitive marketing. In the end, maybe some centers would cease to contribute their data.

But if courage is in scarce supply, so will be the knowledge, and I guess we would have to explain that to Jim Lang. We would have to tell Jim Lang this: "Jim, we'd love to help you about the prom night thing, but we are not the best yet. We would like to study the best places so we can learn from them. But Jim, we are a little stuck, because we can't find out who is the best, because it would be too frightening if we shared the data. Some hospitals would get scared. Some programs would lose market share. Some doctors would get angry. Some lawyers would sue and get rich. Sorry, Jim. We are just not in a position to help. Good luck, Jim. We're right behind you."

You might guess by now that Cincinnati Children's Hospital has refused to give this answer. They found out. Courageously, the CF Foundation helped them after all to get the information they needed, and they are out there right now, asking the humble, courageous question, "Who does this better than we do?" And they will find the answers, and they will help Jim, and Jim's daughter will have a great night at the prom—cross their hearts.

The CF Foundation, kudos to them, is taking on this issue of transparency. They know that ignoring the abundant knowledge in their data is not just wasteful, it is probably immoral. So they are now committed to change, to finding a way to quell the fear, and to connect to the aspiration. It will take some time, but secrecy is no longer an option, and they know it.

Transparency about performance is handmaiden to learning. Improvement requires learning, and secrecy paralyzes learning. It is time for this nation to commit to public measurement and reporting on the quality characteristics of the health care organizations that serve it, not for the purpose of increasing fear, selection, or even accountability. Frankly, I could care less about accountability. I want us to have the courage to show our results for one reason above all others: to help Maria Britto, Jim Acton, and Terri Schindler help Jim Lang make sure that Alicia gets to the prom.

Let me show you what such courage looks like. Three weeks ago I spoke at Tallahassee Memorial Hospital, where I showed Brian Jarman's scatterplot. I know where Tallahassee Memorial is on that scatterplot, and so does its CEO, Duncan Moore. The news is not so good yet. Tallahassee has a ways to go; its standardized mortality rate is 130. Now, Duncan knew that, and I knew he knew that, but it was not my place to say so in public. In the room were two hundred physicians and board members, and closed-circuit TV broadcasts of my speech were being piped into two other assembly rooms and into every patient room in that hospital.

But Duncan, the CEO, interrupted me. In full view of everyone, he asked me, "What is our mortality rate?" I thought he might not have realized what he was asking for. Maybe he forgot. So I said I would check and tell him later. He said, "No, I've seen the data and you know the answer." And he turned to Winnie Schmeling, who is leading their Pursuing Perfection work, and asked her, in front of everyone, "Winnie, where are we?"

Winnie answered, in front of hundreds of staff and who knows how many patients, "We're at 130." Now Duncan already knew that, like I said. But he asked for it anyway, in full view of his board, his staff, and his patients.

I will never forget that moment. Duncan is too self-effacing to accept it, but I know what I saw: courage, aspiration, respect for knowledge, respect for staff, respect for patients, trust in people, trust in learning, trust in the future, unwillingness to waste, optimism, a sense of abundance—all encapsulated in a single, public deed. It is exactly what we need.

Here is how Duncan closed the meeting. He said, "I want you to remember two numbers today. One is 130, which is where we are. And the other is 80, which is where we are going to be."

Asking who does what we do better than we do it opens a wide front door to learning, but we will never ask if we do not believe in the abundance of knowledge around us. The world is our teacher, but only if we put aside the fear and examine the reality of our own performance—openly, with no secrets, no hiding, no bars. Congratulations, Cincinnati Children's. Congratulations, Tallahassee Memorial.

Congratulations, Duncan Moore. You'd like Paul Batalden, by the way. He's a lunatic too.

Abundance has one more form that I'd like to mention this morning, along with the abundance that our patients, our staff, and our data bring to us. The fourth abundance is really a special version of the third—it's knowledge too, but writ larger. Knowledge from the entire world. Global brains, I call it. Health care needs global brains.

Let's start with the basics. America spends 40 percent more dollars per capita on its health care than the next most expensive nation, and more than twice as much as most. For this glut of funding, it gets nowhere near the top health status in the world—we are maybe tenth or twentieth, depending on how you count it. We are the only developed nation on Earth that does not guarantee health care to its people—the only one. At $5,000 per person per year, we leave 45 million souls without health insurance. At under $3,000 per person per year, the United Kingdom leaves no one out—no one—not even illegal immigrants.

You would think that we'd be curious. If someone showed up at your door and said, "I can get you the same car you have today for 60 percent of the price," wouldn't you be just a little curious? At least about whether the guy should be arrested?

It goes for specific conditions, too. For a few procedures, we are the best on Earth, but not for most. At lower cost—far lower cost— many other nations and health care systems get better end-of-life care, better mental health care, better infant mortality rates, better asthma control, better physical rehabilitation, better primary prevention, and much more comprehensive primary care than we do. In cystic fibrosis outcomes we are not the best in the world. We are number two. Denmark is number one.

That is why I want Cincinnati Children's Hospital to visit Denmark—because I want them to refuse to attach a value of zero to the global information available to them. If the world has something to teach us, why would we not learn?

Paul Batalden says that a visitor from Bosnia a few weeks ago took him aside and whispered to him, "I don't get it. I just can't figure it out. How *do* you spend $1.5 trillion?" Paul's answer was another one of those "Hey There, Georgie Girl" comments. He answered, "It's easy; you just need to make more categories." With enough fragments you can waste almost anything.

We really do need to snap out of it. The entire Western world testifies that there are fine ways to provide health insurance to absolutely everybody while investing less than 60 cents on every dollar we spend today. We need to have the courage and the confidence to figure out how to do that ourselves. To say that we spend 15 percent of our gross domestic product on health care and that *that* is not enough—that *that* is scarcity—is ridiculous. It is dishonest. We have enough. We have plenty. What we lack is not social resources; it is honesty.

Let's celebrate our wealth: The abundance in our patients, their families, and their communities—their experience, dedication, intelligence, and courage. The abundance in our amazing workforce—their pride, dedication, imagination, and courage. The abundance in the knowledge that lies in the very diversity of our achievements—accessible through the transparent, scientific, and courageous study of our own performance and the gaps therein. And the abundance in the lessons we have yet to learn from other nations, who, unlike us, know how to do far more good with far less money.

Let's have an abundance party, where you check the assumption of scarcity at the door or you can't get in.

I have a date in mind to suggest for the party—the abundance party. It's not too far away—May 4, 2008. Let's have a party on Alicia Lang's prom night. We can invite her mom and dad, Mary Kaye and Jim, to come too. They'll be available. Alicia won't really want them hanging around her, after all. She'll be too busy having a really good time.

Notes

1. Covey, S. R. *The Seven Habits of Highly Effective People*. New York: Simon and Schuster, 1990.

2. Hawken, P., Lovins, A., and Lovins, H. *Natural Capitalism: Creating the Next Industrial Revolution*. Boston: Little, Brown, 1999.

About the Author

Donald M. Berwick, MD, MPP, is president, CEO, and cofounder of the Institute for Healthcare Improvement (IHI) in Boston. IHI is a not-for-profit organization dedicated to improving the quality of health care systems through education, research, and demonstration projects, and through fostering collaboration among health care organizations and their leaders. Berwick is a clinical professor of pediatrics and health care policy at the Harvard Medical School. He is also a pediatrician, an associate in pediatrics at Boston's Children's Hospital, and a consultant in pediatrics at Massachusetts General Hospital.

An internationally recognized expert on health care quality, Berwick has published extensively in professional journals in the areas of health care policy, decision analysis, technology assessment, and health care quality improvement.

About the Commentary Authors

Introduction

Frank Davidoff, MD, served on the faculty at the Harvard and University of Connecticut Medical Schools prior to becoming senior vice president for education at the American College of Physicians. Editor emeritus of the *Annals of Internal Medicine*, he now serves as executive editor for the Boston-based Institute for Healthcare Improvement. Davidoff has been the principal investigator of research grants from the National Institutes of Health, the National Fund for Medical Education, the Commonwealth Fund, the Pew Charitable Trust, and the American College of Physicians-American Society for Internal Medicine Foundation. He is a member of the Non-Prescription Drug Advisory Committee of the United States Food and Drug Administration, the board of Physicians for Human Rights, and the editorial board of the journal *Quality and Safety in Health Care*. Davidoff's publications include more than sixty original papers and book chapters, in addition to editorials and commentaries on clinical medicine, medical editing, and the environment of medical practice. He is author of a book of essays, *Who Has Seen a Blood Sugar? Reflections on Medical Education*.

1. Kevin Speaks

Susan Edgman-Levitan, PA, is executive director of the John D. Stoeckle Center for Primary Care Innovation at Massachusetts

General Hospital. She is also Institute for Healthcare Improvement (IHI) Fellow for Patient- and Family-Centered Care. She is a lecturer at Harvard Medical School and was founding president of The Picker Institute. An editor of the books *Through the Patient's Eyes* and *Medicine and Pediatrics*, Edgman-Levitan was also coprincipal investigator on Harvard's Agency for Healthcare Research and Quality-funded five-year Consumer Assessment of Health Plans (CAHPS) project and continues as coprincipal investigator on the CAHPS II study (2002–2007). She has served as cochair of IHI's National Forum and the National Patient Safety Foundation Congress and as chair of the IHI Breakthrough Series Collaborative on Improving Service Quality, and is currently a technical adviser for The Robert Wood Johnson Foundation's national program Pursuing Perfection. She is a board member of several organizations, including Planetree, the National Patient Safety Foundation, and the Foundation for Informed Medical Decision Making. She also serves as a commissioner for the Center for Information Therapy.

2. Buckling Down to Change

Thomas W. Nolan, PhD, is a statistician, author, and consultant. He is cofounder of Associates in Process Improvement, a consulting firm that specializes in the improvement of quality and productivity, and a senior fellow and member of the executive team of the Institute for Healthcare Improvement. Over the past twenty years he has assisted organizations in many different industries in the United States, Canada, and Europe, including health care; professional services such as law, architecture, and environmental consulting; and manufacturing, trucking, and construction. His health care experience includes helping integrated systems, hospitals, and medical practices to accelerate the improvement of quality and the reduction of costs in clinical and administrative services. Nolan is currently codirector, along with Donald Berwick, of the Pursuing Perfection initiative funded by The Robert Wood Johnson Foundation. The year 2000 recipient of the Deming Medal awarded by the American Society for Quality, he is author of three books on improving quality and productivity and he has published articles in a variety of peer-reviewed journals.

3. Quality Comes Home

Brian Jarman, MD, is senior fellow at the Institute for Healthcare Improvement as well as professor emeritus at the Imperial College of Science, Technology and Medicine in London. He is former head of the Department of Primary Care and Population Health Sciences Division at Imperial College and a general practitioner in the United Kingdom. He was a resident in medicine at the Beth Israel Hospital, Boston. Jarman is the developer of the Jarman Index (a measure of the extent to which specific locales are underprivileged and at risk of poorer health outcomes). He was a member of the panel of the Bristol Royal Infirmary Inquiry and is developer of a method of measuring standardized mortality ratios based on hospital data. He is extending this work while in the United States. Jarman is president of the British Medical Association for one year (July 2003 through July 2004).

4. Run to Space

Paul Batalden, MD, is director of Health Care Improvement Leadership Development at the Center for the Evaluative Clinical Sciences at Dartmouth Medical School, and a senior vice president of the Institute for Healthcare Improvement. Both a teacher and student of continuous improvement in health care for the past twenty-five years, he was founding chair of the Institute for Healthcare Improvement's board of directors.

5. Sauerkraut, Sobriety, and the Spread of Change

David H. Gustafson, PhD, is Robert Ratner Professor of Industrial Engineering and Preventive Medicine at the University of Wisconsin, Madison, where he founded the Center for Health Systems Research and Analysis in 1973. He currently directs the National Cancer Institute Center of Excellence in Cancer Communication and The Robert Wood Johnson National Program on Paths to Recovery. His quality management research includes development of computer systems to help organizations in their efforts to implement quality management. Gustafson has developed methodologies to better understand customer needs, organizational change, and sustainability. A member of the Institute for Healthcare Improvement's board of directors for ten years, he currently chairs the board of the eHealth Institute and was recently chair of the federal Science Panel on Interactive Communications in Health.

6. Why the *Vasa* Sank

Robert Waller, MD, is president emeritus of Mayo Foundation and served as its president and CEO from 1988 through 1998. He is a former member of the Institute for Healthcare Improvement's board of directors.

7. Eagles and Weasels

Paul Plsek is president of Paul E. Plsek and Associates and an internationally recognized consultant on improvement and innovation. He is author of dozens of articles and three books: *Quality Improvement Tools*; *Creativity, Innovation and Quality*; and *Edgeware: Insights from Complexity Science for Health Care Leaders*.

8. Escape Fire

Karl E. Weick, PhD, is Rensis Likert Distinguished University Professor of Organizational Behavior and Psychology and professor of psychology at the University of Michigan Business School. He joined the Michigan faculty in 1988 after previous faculty positions at the University of Texas, Cornell University, University of Minnesota, and Purdue University. He is a former editor of the journal *Administrative Science Quarterly* (1977–1985), former associate editor of the journal *Organizational Behavior and Human Performance* (1971–1977), and current topic editor for Human Factors at the journal *Wildfire*. Weick is author of numerous articles and books, including *Sensemaking in Organizations* and *Managing the Unexpected: Assuring High Performance in an Age of Complexity*. His research interests include collective sensemaking under pressure, medical errors, handoffs and transitions in dynamic events, high reliability performance, improvisation, and continuous change.

9. Dirty Words and Magic Spells

Maureen Bisognano is executive vice president and COO at the Institute for Healthcare Improvement (IHI) in Boston, Massachusetts. IHI is a premier integrative force for change in the health care industry, providing strategic vision, proven methodologies, and expert knowledge to health care leaders committed to improving the quality of patient care. Bisognano's career has been dedicated to improving health care. Prior to joining IHI, she was senior vice president of The Juran Institute, where she supported the implementation of total quality management concepts in health care settings. Earlier in her career she implemented a comprehensive hospital-based quality improvement program while serving as CEO of Massachusetts Respiratory Hospital in Braintree, Massachusetts. Bisognano received a B.S. degree from the University of the State of New York and a M.S. degree from Boston University. She has authored articles on medical leadership and has helped scores of health care leaders and organizations improve performance.

10. Every Single One

Howard Hiatt, MD, is senior physician at Brigham and Women's Hospital in Boston, Massachusetts; a member of the Institute for Healthcare Improvement's board of directors; and professor of medicine at Harvard Medical School. Previously he served as physician-chief at Beth Israel Hospital in Boston, and then as dean of the Harvard School of Public Health.

11. Plenty

Vinod K. Sahney, PhD, is senior vice president of planning and strategic development for the Henry Ford Health System in Detroit. He is a founding member and current chair of the board of directors of the Institute for Healthcare Improvement. Sahney is also a member of both the Institute of Medicine and the National Academy of Engineering. For the past twenty-seven years he has been a visiting faculty member of executive programs at Harvard University School of Public Health.

Index